Establishing Effective Patient Navigation Programs in Oncology

PROCEEDINGS OF A WORKSHOP

Margie Patlak, Cyndi Trang, and Sharyl J. Nass, *Rapporteurs*

National Cancer Policy Forum

Board on Health Care Services

Health and Medicine Division

The National Academies of
SCIENCES · ENGINEERING · MEDICINE

THE NATIONAL ACADEMIES PRESS
Washington, DC
www.nap.edu

THE NATIONAL ACADEMIES PRESS 500 Fifth Street, NW Washington, DC 20001

This activity was supported by Contract No. 200-2011-38807 (Task Order No. 0061) and Contract No. HHSN263201200074I (Task Order No. HHSN26300120) with the Centers for Disease Control and Prevention and the National Cancer Institute/National Institutes of Health, respectively, and by the American Association for Cancer Research, American Cancer Society, American College of Radiology, American Society of Clinical Oncology, American Society of Hematology, Association of American Cancer Institutes, Bristol-Myers Squibb, Cancer Support Community, CEO Roundtable on Cancer, Flatiron Health, Helsinn Therapeutics (U.S.), Inc., LIVESTRONG Foundation, Merck, National Comprehensive Cancer Network, Novartis Oncology, Oncology Nursing Society, and Pfizer Inc. Any opinions, findings, conclusions, or recommendations expressed in this publication do not necessarily reflect the views of any organization or agency that provided support for the project.

International Standard Book Number-13: 978-0-309-47454-2
International Standard Book Number-10: 0-309-47454-X
Digital Object Identifier: https://doi.org/10.17226/25073

Additional copies of this publication are available for sale from the National Academies Press, 500 Fifth Street, NW, Keck 360, Washington, DC 20001; (800) 624-6242 or (202) 334-3313; http://www.nap.edu.

Printed in the United States of America

Suggested citation: National Academies of Sciences, Engineering, and Medicine. 2018. *Establishing effective patient navigation programs in oncology: Proceedings of a workshop.* Washington, DC: The National Academies Press. doi: https://doi.org/10.17226/25073.

The National Academies of
SCIENCES · ENGINEERING · MEDICINE

The **National Academy of Sciences** was established in 1863 by an Act of Congress, signed by President Lincoln, as a private, nongovernmental institution to advise the nation on issues related to science and technology. Members are elected by their peers for outstanding contributions to research. Dr. Marcia McNutt is president.

The **National Academy of Engineering** was established in 1964 under the charter of the National Academy of Sciences to bring the practices of engineering to advising the nation. Members are elected by their peers for extraordinary contributions to engineering. Dr. C. D. Mote, Jr., is president.

The **National Academy of Medicine** (formerly the Institute of Medicine) was established in 1970 under the charter of the National Academy of Sciences to advise the nation on medical and health issues. Members are elected by their peers for distinguished contributions to medicine and health. Dr. Victor J. Dzau is president.

The three Academies work together as the **National Academies of Sciences, Engineering, and Medicine** to provide independent, objective analysis and advice to the nation and conduct other activities to solve complex problems and inform public policy decisions. The National Academies also encourage education and research, recognize outstanding contributions to knowledge, and increase public understanding in matters of science, engineering, and medicine.

Learn more about the National Academies of Sciences, Engineering, and Medicine at **www.nationalacademies.org.**

The National Academies of

SCIENCES • ENGINEERING • MEDICINE

Consensus Study Reports published by the National Academies of Sciences, Engineering, and Medicine document the evidence-based consensus on the study's statement of task by an authoring committee of experts. Reports typically include findings, conclusions, and recommendations based on information gathered by the committee and the committee's deliberations. Each report has been subjected to a rigorous and independent peer-review process and it represents the position of the National Academies on the statement of task.

Proceedings published by the National Academies of Sciences, Engineering, and Medicine chronicle the presentations and discussions at a workshop, symposium, or other event convened by the National Academies. The statements and opinions contained in proceedings are those of the participants and are not endorsed by other participants, the planning committee, or the National Academies.

For information about other products and activities of the National Academies, please visit www.nationalacademies.org/about/whatwedo.

WORKSHOP PLANNING COMMITTEE[1]

LISA KENNEDY SHELDON (*Co-Chair*), Chief Clinical Officer, Oncology Nursing Society

LAWRENCE N. SHULMAN (*Co-Chair*), Professor of Medicine, Deputy Director for Clinical Services, and Director, Center for Global Cancer Medicine, Abramson Cancer Center, University of Pennsylvania

LUCILE L. ADAMS-CAMPBELL, Professor of Oncology, Associate Director for Minority Health and Health Disparities Research, Georgetown University Lombardi Cancer Center

KAREN BASEN-ENGQUIST, Annie Laurie Howard Research Distinguished Professor, Professor of Behavioral Science, and Director, Center for Energy Balance in Cancer Prevention and Survivorship, The University of Texas MD Anderson Cancer Center

DARCY BURBAGE, Supportive and Palliative Care Nurse Navigator, Helen F. Graham Cancer Center & Research Institute, Christiana Care Health System

CYNTHIA CANTRIL, Director, Cancer Support Services and Patient Navigation, Sutter Pacific Medical Foundation

EFRÉN J. FLORES, Radiologist, Director, Community Health Improvement, Department of Radiology, Massachusetts General Hospital

ELIZABETH FRANKLIN, Senior Director, Policy and Advocacy, Cancer Support Community

LORI HOFFMAN HŌGG, Veterans Health Administration National Oncology Clinical Advisor and Program Manager, Prevention Policy, Department of Veterans Affairs

RONALD M. KLINE, Medical Officer, Patient Care Models Group, Center for Medicare & Medicaid Innovation, Centers for Medicare & Medicaid Services

ADITI NARAYAN, Senior Manager, Patient Support and Research, LIVESTRONG Foundation

[1] The National Academies of Sciences, Engineering, and Medicine's planning committees are solely responsible for organizing the workshop, identifying topics, and choosing speakers. The responsibility for the published Proceedings of a Workshop rests with the workshop rapporteurs and the institution.

MANDI PRATT-CHAPMAN, Associate Center Director, Patient-Centered Initiatives and Health Equity, George Washington Cancer Center

ELIZABETH ROHAN, Health Scientist, Division of Cancer Prevention and Control, Centers for Disease Control and Prevention

KIRSTEN SLOAN, Vice President, Health Policy, American Cancer Society Cancer Action Network

GEORGE J. WEINER, C.E. Block Chair of Cancer Research, Professor of Internal Medicine, and Director, Holden Comprehensive Cancer Center, The University of Iowa

WENDY A. WOODWARD, Associate Professor and Service Chief, Clinical Breast Radiation, Department of Radiation Oncology, The University of Texas MD Anderson Cancer Center

Project Staff

ERIN BALOGH, Senior Program Officer

NATALIE LUBIN, Senior Program Assistant

KELLY SINGEL, Mirzayan Science and Technology Policy Fellow (January 2018–April 2018)

CYNDI TRANG, Research Assistant

SHARYL J. NASS, Director, National Cancer Policy Forum and Board on Health Care Services

NATIONAL CANCER POLICY FORUM[1]

EDWARD J. BENZ, JR. (*Chair*), President and Chief Executive Officer Emeritus, Dana-Farber Cancer Institute; Richard and Susan Smith Distinguished Professor of Medicine, Genetics and Pediatrics, Harvard Medical School

AMY P. ABERNETHY, Chief Medical Officer, Chief Scientific Officer, and Senior Vice President, Oncology, Flatiron Health

LUCILE L. ADAMS-CAMPBELL, Professor of Oncology, Associate Director for Minority Health and Health Disparities Research, Georgetown University Lombardi Cancer Center

GARNET L. ANDERSON, Senior Vice President and Director, Public Health Sciences Division, Fred Hutchinson Cancer Research Center; Affiliate Professor, Department of Biostatistics, University of Washington

KENNETH ANDERSON, Kraft Family Professor of Medicine, American Cancer Society Clinical Research Director, Jerome Lipper Multiple Myeloma Center, Harvard Medical School, Dana-Farber Cancer Institute

KAREN BASEN-ENGQUIST, Annie Laurie Howard Research Distinguished Professor, Professor of Behavioral Science, and Director, Center for Energy Balance in Cancer Prevention and Survivorship, The University of Texas MD Anderson Cancer Center

CATHY J. BRADLEY, Associate Director, Cancer Prevention and Control, University of Colorado Cancer Center

OTIS W. BRAWLEY, Chief Medical Officer, American Cancer Society

ROBERT W. CARLSON, Chief Executive Officer, National Comprehensive Cancer Network

CHRISTOPHER R. COGLE, Professor of Medicine, Pierre Chagnon Professor of Stem Cell Biology and Bone Marrow Transplant, University of Florida; Scholar in Clinical Research, Leukemia & Lymphoma Society

[1] The National Academies of Sciences, Engineering, and Medicine's forums and roundtables do not issue, review, or approve individual documents. The responsibility for the published Proceedings of a Workshop rests with the workshop rapporteurs and the institution.

NANCY E. DAVIDSON, President and Executive Director, Seattle Cancer Care Alliance; Senior Vice President, Director, and Full Member, Clinical Research Division, Fred Hutchinson Cancer Research Center; Head, Department of Medicine, Division of Medical Oncology, University of Washington

GEORGE D. DEMETRI, Professor of Medicine and Director, Ludwig Center, Harvard Medical School; Senior Vice President for Experimental Therapeutics, Dana-Farber Cancer Institute; Associate Director for Clinical Sciences, Dana-Farber/Harvard Cancer Center

JAMES H. DOROSHOW, Deputy Director for Clinical and Translational Research, National Cancer Institute

NICOLE F. DOWLING, Associate Director, Division of Cancer Prevention and Control, Centers for Disease Control and Prevention

SCOT W. EBBINGHAUS, Vice President and Therapeutic Area Head, Oncology Clinical Research, Merck Research Laboratories

KOJO S. J. ELENITOBA-JOHNSON, Professor, Perelman School of Medicine; Director, Center for Personalized Diagnostics and Division of Precision and Computational Diagnostics, University of Pennsylvania

STANTON L. GERSON, President, Association of American Cancer Institutes; Director, Case Comprehensive Cancer Center; Professor of Hematological Oncology, Case Western Reserve University; Director, University Hospitals Seidman Cancer Center

LORI HOFFMAN HŌGG, Veterans Health Administration National Oncology Clinical Advisor and Program Manager, Prevention Policy, Department of Veterans Affairs

LINDA HOUSE, President, Cancer Support Community

HEDVIG HRICAK, Chair, Department of Radiology, Memorial Sloan Kettering Cancer Center

LISA KENNEDY SHELDON, Chief Clinical Officer, Oncology Nursing Society

SAMIR N. KHLEIF, Director, Loop Immuno-Oncology Lab, Biomedical Scholar, and Professor of Oncology, Lombardi Comprehensive Cancer Center, Georgetown University Medical Center

RONALD M. KLINE, Medical Officer, Patient Care Models Group, Center for Medicare & Medicaid Innovation, Centers for Medicare & Medicaid Services

LEE M. KRUG, Disease Area Head, Lung and Head & Neck Cancer, Immuno-Oncology, Bristol-Myers Squibb

MICHELLE M. LE BEAU, Arthur and Marian Edelstein Professor of Medicine and Director, The University of Chicago Comprehensive Cancer Center

MIA LEVY, Director, Cancer Health Informatics and Strategy; Ingram Associate Professor of Cancer Research; Associate Professor of Biomedical Informatics and Medicine, Vanderbilt-Ingram Cancer Center

MARTIN J. MURPHY, Chief Executive Officer, CEO Roundtable on Cancer

RICHARD PAZDUR, Director, Oncology Center of Excellence; Acting Director, Office of Hematology and Oncology Products, Food and Drug Administration

MACE L. ROTHENBERG, Chief Development Officer, Oncology, Pfizer Global Product Development, Pfizer Inc.

RICHARD L. SCHILSKY, Senior Vice President and Chief Medical Officer, American Society of Clinical Oncology

DEBORAH SCHRAG, Chief, Division of Population Sciences, Professor of Medicine, Department of Medical Oncology, Harvard Medical School, Dana-Farber Cancer Institute

LAWRENCE N. SHULMAN, Professor of Medicine, Deputy Director for Clinical Services, and Director, Center for Global Cancer Medicine, Abramson Cancer Center, University of Pennsylvania

DAN THEODORESCU, Paul A. Bunn, Jr. Endowed Chair in Cancer Research, Professor of Surgery and Pharmacology, and Director, University of Colorado Cancer Center

VERENA VOELTER, Head, United States Oncology Clinical Development & Medical Affairs, Novartis Pharmaceuticals Corporation

GEORGE J. WEINER, C.E. Block Chair of Cancer Research, Professor of Internal Medicine, and Director, Holden Comprehensive Cancer Center, The University of Iowa

ROBERT A. WINN, Associate Vice Chancellor, Community Based-Practice; Professor of Medicine, Division of Pulmonary and Critical Care Medicine, University of Illinois at Chicago; Director, University of Illinois Health Cancer Center

National Cancer Policy Forum Staff

ERIN BALOGH, Senior Program Officer
PATRICK BURKE, Financial Officer
NATALIE LUBIN, Senior Program Assistant
KELLY SINGEL, Mirzayan Science and Technology Policy Fellow (January 2018–April 2018)
CYNDI TRANG, Research Assistant
SHARYL J. NASS, Director, National Cancer Policy Forum and Board on Health Care Services

Reviewers

This Proceedings of a Workshop was reviewed in draft form by individuals chosen for their diverse perspectives and technical expertise. The purpose of this independent review is to provide candid and critical comments that will assist the National Academies of Sciences, Engineering, and Medicine in making each published proceedings as sound as possible and to ensure that it meets the institutional standards for quality, objectivity, evidence, and responsiveness to the charge. The review comments and draft manuscript remain confidential to protect the integrity of the process.

We thank the following individuals for their review of this proceedings:

ETHAN BASCH, University of North Carolina at Chapel Hill
LINDA HORN, Patient Advocate and Cancer Survivor
RAYMOND OSAROGIAGBON, Baptist Cancer Center
ANGIE PATTERSON, Georgia Center for Oncology Research and Education
MELISSA SIMON, Northwestern University Feinberg School of Medicine

Although the reviewers listed above provided many constructive comments and suggestions, they were not asked to endorse the content of the proceedings nor did they see the final draft before its release. The review of this proceedings was overseen by **PATRICK DeLEON,** Uniformed

Services University of the Health Sciences. He was responsible for making certain that an independent examination of this proceedings was carried out in accordance with standards of the National Academies and that all review comments were carefully considered. Responsibility for the final content rests entirely with the rapporteurs and the National Academies.

Acknowledgments

Support from the many sponsors of the National Academies of Sciences, Engineering, and Medicine's National Cancer Policy Forum is crucial to the work of the forum. Federal sponsors include the Centers for Disease Control and Prevention and the National Cancer Institute/National Institutes of Health. Non-federal sponsors include the American Association for Cancer Research, American Cancer Society, American College of Radiology, American Society of Clinical Oncology, American Society of Hematology, Association of American Cancer Institutes, Bristol-Myers Squibb, Cancer Support Community, CEO Roundtable on Cancer, Flatiron Health, Helsinn Therapeutics (U.S.), Inc., LIVESTRONG Foundation, Merck, National Comprehensive Cancer Network, Novartis Oncology, Oncology Nursing Society, and Pfizer Inc.

The forum wishes to express its gratitude to the expert speakers whose presentations helped further the dialogue and advance progress in improving patient navigation for patients with cancer. The forum also wishes to thank the members of the planning committee for their work in developing an excellent workshop agenda.

Contents

Boxes, Figures, and Table

BOXES

FIGURES

TABLE

Acronyms and Abbreviations

ACA	Patient Protection and Affordable Care Act
ACS	American Cancer Society
AONN+	Academy of Oncology Nurse & Patient Navigators
CMS	Centers for Medicare & Medicaid Services
CoC	Commission on Cancer
CORE	Center for Oncology Research and Education
CPNG	Cancer Patient Navigators of Georgia
DPNC	DuPage Patient Navigation Collaborative
EHR	electronic health record
GATE	Generation and Translation of Evidence
HIV	human immunodeficiency virus
HRSA	Health Resources and Services Administration
MGH	Massachusetts General Hospital
NCI	National Cancer Institute
NNRT	National Navigation Roundtable

OCM	Oncology Care Model
ONS	Oncology Nursing Society
PACE	presenting information, asking questions, checking for understanding, and expressing concerns
PCCP	Patient Care Connect Program
PN-BOT	Patient Navigation Barriers and Outcomes Tool
PNRP	Patient Navigation Research Program
PSA	prostate-specific antigen
REDCap	Research Electronic Data Capture
TEAM	Together-Equitable-Accessible-Meaningful
TRIP	Translating Research Into Practice
WWC	Women's Wellness Connection

Proceedings of a Workshop

INTRODUCTION[1]

Delivering high-quality cancer care to all patients presents numerous challenges, including difficulties with care coordination and access. Patient navigation "is a community-based service delivery intervention designed to promote access to timely diagnosis and treatment of cancer and other chronic diseases by eliminating barriers to care" (Freeman and Rodriguez, 2011). Patient navigation has often been proposed and implemented to address these challenges. Harold P. Freeman, chief executive officer, president, and founder of the Harold P. Freeman Patient Navigation Institute, developed the patient navigation concept and created the first cancer-specific navigation program in 1990. The program's main objective is to remove barriers to cancer care for underserved patients in Harlem. Since then, numerous patient navigation programs have been developed with different approaches and goals for various patient populations, and a substantial body of scientific evidence from many studies on the benefits

[1] The planning committee's role was limited to planning the workshop, and the Proceedings of a Workshop was prepared by the workshop rapporteurs as a factual summary of what occurred at the workshop. Statements, recommendations, and opinions expressed are those of individual presenters and participants, and are not necessarily endorsed or verified by the National Academies of Sciences, Engineering, and Medicine, and they should not be construed as reflecting any group consensus.

of navigation has been generated (see the section on Evidence on Patient Navigation).

Although many navigation programs focus on improving cancer screening rates and early detection, some are also used to improve timely cancer diagnosis and treatment, clinical trial enrollment, and care transitions. Some navigation services continue into long-term survivorship care as well. Most navigation programs help patients overcome barriers to care, such as challenges with health literacy or fluency in the English language affecting comprehension of diagnosis and treatment; lack of transportation; or insufficient insurance coverage. Patient navigators also strive to build and strengthen the communications and relationships between patients and health care professionals while addressing psychosocial concerns for the patient and family. Another common role of navigators is to close the gaps in the health care system by tracking patient care and ensuring handoffs from one care provider to another.

A fundamental debate revolves around how to define patient navigation and what patient navigation programs should entail, as well as who should provide navigation services. Early efforts relied primarily on non-clinicians. Currently, most navigators are nurses or community health workers, but programs may also include case managers, social workers, tumor registrars, or cancer patient peers who serve as volunteers. Many programs emphasize the need to train navigators in cultural and linguistic aspects relevant to the population being served, as race/ethnicity and language concordance between navigator and patient has been linked to improved health care delivery.

Unresolved questions include where patient navigation programs should be deployed and which patients should be prioritized to receive navigation services when resources are limited. Patient navigation systems are often implemented as an attempt to address socioeconomic disparities in care delivery. Therefore, many interventions have been clustered in predominantly minority and economically underserved areas, often in urban cancer centers. However, navigation programs often go beyond poor and underserved patients to aid all patients. Experts also continue to debate whether patient navigation should be proactive or reactive, and who benefits most from using navigation programs, particularly with regard to ongoing concerns about the cost and value of care.

To address these issues and facilitate discussions on how to improve navigation services for patients with cancer, the National Cancer Policy Forum of the National Academies of Sciences, Engineering, and Medicine held a workshop on Establishing Effective Patient Navigation Programs in Oncology in Washington, DC, on November 13 and 14, 2017. At this workshop, a broad range of experts and stakeholders, including clinicians, navigators, researchers, and patients, provided an overview of patient navigation programs and explored:

- Which patients need navigation and who should serve as navigators;
- The benefits of navigation and current gaps in the evidence base;
- Patient navigation models and lessons learned when implementing navigation programs;
- Standards, training, and certification for patient navigation;
- Policy challenges and opportunities; and
- Recent policy initiatives.

A number of workshop participants also suggested numerous changes to improve navigation services for patients with cancer (see Box 1). This proceedings is a summary of the presentations and discussions at the

BOX 1
Suggestions from Individual Workshop Participants to Improve Patient Navigation Programs in Oncology

Providing Effective Navigation Services Throughout the Oncology Care Continuum

- Establish navigation strategies for all stages of care (e.g., prevention and screening, diagnosis, treatment, survivorship care, and end-of-life care). (Freeman, Paskett, Shulman)
- Enhance collaboration among the members of multidisciplinary care teams, from navigators to physicians. (Fitzpatrick, Freeman, Pratt-Chapman, Valania)
- Screen patients to identify those with the greatest need of navigation services. (Buescher, Freeman, Shulman, Valania)
- Foster self-care management by patients receiving navigation services. (Meneses)
- Empower patients and maximize uptake of navigation services by enhancing convenience of services. (Narayan)
- Identify and address evidence gaps for patient navigation (e.g., impact on palliative care, cancers other than breast). (Paskett, Shulman)

continued

BOX 1 Continued

Improving Education for Patient Navigation

- Standardize training and certification for all navigators, regardless of professional role. (Blackley, Horn, Nevidjon, Paskett, Pratt-Chapman, Shulman)
- Define the roles, responsibilities, and boundaries of the navigator within the care team. (Burbage, Freeman, Valania)
- Clarify different roles of navigators with different professional backgrounds. (Paskett, Pratt-Chapman, Melissa Simon)
- Clarify expectations and best practices for interactions with patients and among team members. (Pratt-Chapman)
- Inform navigators about resources in the community so they can refer patients. (Pratt-Chapman, Valania)
- Recruit navigators with important traits and capabilities for the role, including ability to organize, multitask, and reprioritize workflow. (Burbage, Valania)

Coordinating and Managing Patient Navigation Teams

- Assign a navigation coordinator who is responsible for overseeing all phases of navigation activity within a given health care system. (Freeman)
- Establish operational procedures and supports, with clear policies. (Oo, Pratt-Chapman, Shulman, Valania)
- Create streamlined care maps for common problems. (Pratt-Chapman)
- Deploy telehealth tools, such as online patient portals, to enable patient communication with care providers, including virtual visits. (Burbage, Tony Burns, Pratt-Chapman)
- Consider adding patient-reported outcomes for communication between patients and navigators for symptom monitoring. (Kline, Paskett, Shulman, Melissa Simon)
- Enhance dialogue, information sharing, and transparency across the health care team. (Cantril, Pratt-Chapman)

Assessing Needs and Resources for Successful Patient Navigation

- Delineate the population(s) a program would serve, conduct a community health needs assessment, and identify gaps or bottlenecks in the services provided. (Blackley, Lathan, Pratt-Chapman, Valania)
- Tailor programs, including navigator training, to fit the culture of the communities that will use them. (Blackley, Cantril, Oo, Pratt-Chapman, Melissa Simon)
- Incorporate community perspectives on pain management, palliative care, and end-of-life care. (Fischer)

- Ask patients, clinicians, and other stakeholders what would be most helpful when developing a new navigation program. (Burbage)
- Consider the complexities of clinical care and health care systems, as well as the impact of a program on care providers. (Melissa Simon)
- Create a national clearinghouse to disseminate navigation resources. (Burbage, Cantril, Pratt-Chapman)
- Determine the skills required in different phases of navigation. (Freeman)

Assessing Patient Navigation Programs

- Establish a system at the onset of a navigation program for tracking metrics. (Blackley, Buescher, Shulman)
- Specify how metrics will be used to improve the program. (Melissa Simon, Pratt-Chapman)
- Incorporate process measures (e.g., timeliness of care, use of distress screening or pain assessments at every visit, with appropriate follow-up). (Buescher)
- Incorporate patient-centered metrics (e.g., treatment adherence, patient-reported outcomes, patient satisfaction), in addition to traditional patient outcomes like mortality. (Pratt-Chapman)
- Incorporate analyses of cost and return on investment (e.g., missed appointments, unplanned hospital admissions, out-migration to another health care system). (Buescher, Evans, Osarogiagbon, Paskett, Shulman)
- Communicate with navigators, patient advisory councils, and clinicians about what is working within the navigation program and what needs to be improved. (Burbage)
- Develop standards for structuring navigation programs to maximize outcomes. (Buescher, Shulman, Melissa Simon)

Addressing Policy Challenges and Opportunities for Making Navigation Affordable

- Sustain patient navigation using different models and payment structures (e.g., bundled and value-based payments). (Kline, Miller, Paskett, Pratt-Chapman, Shulman)
- Leverage resources for navigation by arranging group visits for patients. (Burbage)
- Target navigation resources to patients with the greatest needs to reduce disparities. (Freeman, Pratt-Chapman)
- Engage public health departments to make patient navigation a statewide priority. (Horn, McCracken, Rohan, Greg Simon)

workshop. The workshop statement of task and agenda can be found in Appendixes A and B, respectively. The webcast and speakers' presentations have been archived online.[2]

HISTORY OF PATIENT NAVIGATION

Freeman noted that when he first came to work as a surgeon at a hospital in Harlem, he "wanted to cut cancer out of Harlem." But in the breast clinic there, he cared for many women who had visible tumors that were sometimes so advanced they were ulcerated at the time of diagnosis. This led him to appreciate the need to facilitate early detection via breast cancer screening, and he made it possible for women to undergo such screening free of charge. But then he realized that many women who were screened were dropping out of their medical care and lost to follow-up. As president of the American Cancer Society (ACS) in 1989, Freeman held hearings in seven American cities on what happens to poor people who have cancer. He realized that being poor and having cancer was "a lethal combination" because poor people of any ethnic group face barriers when they attempt to traverse the complex health care system in the United States. He observed that cancer "was not limited to being a surgery problem or medical problem." The health disparities he observed were deeply rooted in the socioeconomic circumstances in poor communities, which could include

- inadequate physical and social environment;
- inadequate information and knowledge;
- risk-promoting lifestyle, attitude, and/or behavior; and
- diminished access to health care (Freeman, 1989).

Based on these hearings, a report by the ACS concluded that poor people who encounter barriers in seeking diagnosis or treatment for cancer are fatalistic about their prognosis (ACS, 1989). The report also concluded that current cancer education programs were culturally insensitive and irrelevant to many poor people, and that people in poverty and their families often had to make extraordinary and personal sacrifices to obtain and pay for their cancer care. Consequently, poor people experienced more pain and suffering from late-stage cancers.

---

[2] See http://www.nationalacademies.org/hmd/Activities/Disease/NCPF/2017-NOV-13.aspx (accessed February 26, 2018).

These findings led Freeman to devise the concept of patient navigation "because if people cannot get into and through a complex system, I thought maybe navigation would help," he said. In 1990, he started a patient navigation system at Harlem Hospital that used laypeople to help cancer patients navigate the health care system. These navigators guided breast cancer patients from the time of an abnormal finding at a free screening clinic through their diagnosis and treatment. Such navigators helped the patients understand what the clinicians told them, tried to alleviate any fear or mistrust they might have of their clinicians, and tried to overcome any financial or other barriers to receiving the treatments patients required.

In 1995, Freeman published his first paper on patient navigation (Freeman et al., 1995), and by 2003, he had demonstrated a significant improvement in the outcomes for women with breast cancer who were treated at Harlem Hospital (Freeman and Wasfie, 1989; Oluwole et al., 2003). Before women had access to breast cancer screening and patient navigation, the 5-year survival rate for breast cancer was 39 percent; only 6 percent of women were diagnosed with Stage I disease, while 49 percent were diagnosed with late-stage breast cancer. After 5 years of instituting free breast cancer screening combined with patient navigation, the 5-year survival rate had risen to 70 percent, and the percentage of women with Stage I disease at diagnosis had risen to 41 percent.

Encouraged by these results, in 2004 the National Cancer Institute (NCI) funded nine patient navigator demonstration sites, said Freeman. Then in 2005, Congress passed the Patient Navigator Outreach and Chronic Disease Prevention Act,[3] which authorized the Secretary of Health and Human Services to fund grants through 2010 for the development of patient navigator programs. A total of $25 million was awarded over 5 years for patient navigator programs through the Community Health Centers and the Office of Rural Health Policy of the Health Resources and Services Administration (HRSA), the NCI, and the Indian Health Service. The overall purpose of the funding was to determine whether patient navigators help to reduce barriers to access to care and improve health care outcomes in underserved patient populations (Urrea, 2009).

In 2005, the NCI funded the Patient Navigation Research Program (PNRP). The PNRP was designed to determine whether patient navigation

[3] See https://www.congress.gov/congressional-report/109th-congress/house-report/104/1 (accessed February 28, 2018).

reduced the time from the point of identifying an abnormal cancer-related finding to the point of diagnosis. The weight of evidence of this 5-year study indicated that patient navigation can reduce the time from abnormal finding to diagnosis in breast, colorectal, cervix, and prostate cancers (Freeman, 2012).

In 2006, the Centers for Medicare & Medicaid Services (CMS) funded six patient navigation demonstration sites, and in 2008 HRSA funded six more demonstration sites, said Freeman. Passage of the Patient Protection and Affordable Care Act (ACA) in 2010 required states to use patient navigators to facilitate access to health insurance and renewed the Patient Navigator Outreach and Chronic Disease Prevention Act. By 2012, the American College of Surgeons Commission on Cancer (CoC) mandated that patient navigation be a standard of care for the more than 1,500 cancer centers accredited by the CoC.

BOX 2
Disparities in Cancer Care

Harold P. Freeman, chief executive officer, president, and founder of the Harold P. Freeman Patient Navigation Institute, noted that nearly 30 million Americans do not have health insurance (Zammitti et al., 2017), which can make it difficult for patients to get cutting-edge cancer treatments (Freeman, 2001). "This discovery-to-delivery disconnect is a key determinant of the unequal burden of cancer," he said.

Kris McCracken, program coordinator of the Women's Wellness Connection at the Colorado Department of Public Health and Environment, added, "Health is not the same thing as health care. A person's community and environment are typically the largest determinants of a person's health. If you are poor, a person of color, lacking education, or living in a rural area, you are not as likely to live as long or as well as other Americans."

Melissa Simon, professor and vice chair of clinical research in the department of obstetrics and gynecology at Northwestern University Feinberg School of Medicine and the Robert H. Lurie Comprehensive Cancer Center, pointed out that health inequities are due to a system that unfairly gives advantages or disadvantages to certain individuals and communities. Rectifying health inequities requires recognition that some

WHY PATIENT NAVIGATION?

Several workshop participants further delineated the importance of patient navigation in helping patients overcome barriers to their health care. Electra Paskett, program leader of the Cancer Control Program at The Ohio State University, pointed out that barriers to care can be at the system, clinician, or patient level. By addressing those barriers, "patient navigators will get patients into the health care system faster . . . and the cancers will be treated earlier," she said.

Many speakers focused on the barriers that can contribute to health disparities (see Box 2). Melissa Simon, professor and vice chair of clinical research in the department of obstetrics and gynecology at the Northwestern University Feinberg School of Medicine and the Robert H. Lurie Comprehensive Cancer Center, noted that a system-level barrier that contributes to health care disparities among patients with breast cancer is public policy

people or communities need more support than others, and providing that extra support with navigation. It is akin to providing a taller stool to a shorter person and vice versa so that all can reach apples in an apple orchard, she noted.

She said several studies have demonstrated health inequities in cancer care and outcomes. For example, breast cancer mortality among African American women in New York City, Chicago, or the United States in general has been reported to be 27, 62, or 41 percent greater, respectively, than that of white women (Hirschman et al., 2007; Hunt et al., 2014; Whitman et al., 2011). Stacy Fischer, associate professor at the University of Colorado School of Medicine, said one study in New York City found that pharmacies located in neighborhoods predominantly populated by people of color were significantly less likely to have adequate opioid stocks to treat cancer patients in pain compared with those in white neighborhoods (Morrison et al., 2000). Christopher Lathan, medical director at the Dana-Farber Cancer Institute at St. Elizabeth's Medical Center, added that cancer mortality varies significantly by ethnicity in Boston (Boston Public Health Commission, 2013) and noted that there are also health inequities among people who speak languages other than English; the lesbian, gay, bisexual, and transgender community; those with a low socioeconomic status; and the rural poor. "It is not just about race," he stressed.

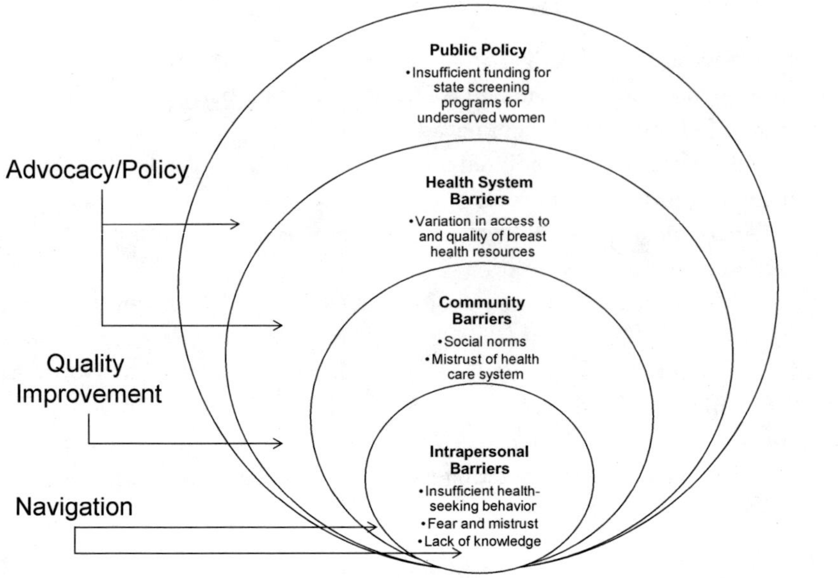

FIGURE 1 Structural elements of the ecology of breast cancer disparities and strategies to address them.
SOURCE: Melissa Simon presentation, November 13, 2017.

that does not ensure adequate funding for state screening programs and public health clinics for underserved populations.

She added that at the community and patient levels, there may be barriers due to fear and mistrust of the health care system. These barriers and a lack of medical knowledge may prevent patients from seeking medical care (see Figure 1). Freeman stressed that the main barriers to cancer care are financial limitations, communication difficulties, health care system bureaucracies, and fear and distrust of the medical community.

Addressing the Impact of Poverty on Cancer Care

Freeman stressed that the effects of poverty are extensive, including inadequate physical and social environments, information, knowledge, and diminished access to health care, as well as risk-promoting lifestyles, attitudes, and behaviors, all of which decrease cancer survival (Freeman, 1989). Nina Miller, manager of CoC cancer liaison initiatives, said a review of the 2017 CoC accreditation survey results found that health care costs and lack of insurance coverage were among the top patient barriers cited.

Christine Valania, oncology social worker and patient navigator for Geisinger Medical Center Cancer Services, said a major care barrier related to poverty is a lack of adequate health insurance that can leave patients with thousands of dollars in out-of-pocket expenses they cannot afford. "They are freaking out and questioning whether they should even move forward with treatment. This is more than knowing insurance. This is really about helping folks find the comfort and understanding that we will help them figure this out," she said. Karen Meneses, professor and associate dean at The University of Alabama at Birmingham, concurred that in her patient population, "Issues regarding payment and the extensive out-of-pocket costs incurred by patients are very much at the front of our thoughts, as well as the travel costs."

Paskett pointed out that large medical bills can lead to patients being evicted from an apartment or having the heat turned off at a residence, both of which can impede their cancer care. As Valania noted, "When people do not have their basic needs met, they are unable to achieve even the smallest tasks. If they do not have food, a place to live, or a ride, they are not coming back for chemo."

Just an inability to afford transportation to a treatment center can hamper the delivery of cancer care, Freeman noted, let alone a lack of health insurance. He emphasized that "no person should die from cancer because they are poor. Let's navigate our population."

Communication and Education

Inadequate communication between clinician and patient is a common barrier to cancer care that patient navigators can address, as several speakers pointed out, and can be due to a patient's lack of fluency in English, health literacy, or self-efficacy, or to insensitivity on the part of clinicians. Melissa Simon noted that some patients may also lack financial literacy. "There are many realms of literacy [that] we have to be aware of and incorporate those into our work," she said.

Reminder letters for appointments are usually in English, which can limit their usefulness for patients who only speak Spanish, said Paskett. Immigrants may also need patient navigators to teach them the skills to navigate the health care system on their own. For example, when a patient navigator takes a patient to an appointment at the main campus of

Massachusetts General Hospital (MGH), the navigator shows the patient where to check in, said Sarah Oo, director of community health improvement at the MGH Chelsea HealthCare Center. "It is guiding and teaching so that the patients feel comfortable that they can do it the next time on their own. We try to build the patients' self-efficacy and their confidence in taking care of their own health," said Oo. Burbage and Meneses agreed that navigators try to empower patients to advocate for themselves, and to foster self-care management. "It is not 'I am sick and you take care of me,' but 'I am sick and how can I and my family better learn how to take care of me?'" But Greg Simon, president of the Biden Cancer Initiative, added that communication will not be adequate "if we do not balance the power between the medical system and the patients so that the patients use their voice because they know it will be heard."

Darcy Burbage, supportive and palliative care nurse navigator at the Christiana Care Health System, also emphasized the roles of navigators in providing patient education, especially with regard to symptom management, available resources, and clinical trials. Sometimes patient navigators will ask clinicians to explain things better to patients who are having trouble understanding their medical situation and options, she said.

Christopher Lathan, medical director at the Dana-Farber Cancer Institute at St. Elizabeth's Medical Center, added that his facility has nurse navigators conduct literacy checks on patients because many patients do not like to admit that they are functionally illiterate. "About 60 percent of what we are doing is trying to figure out the best way to explain things to this patient, which is not necessarily the same as to another patient," he said. Paskett noted that patient navigators at her facility ask patients what they understand about their diagnosis and treatment plan, what their questions are, and then try to bridge communication between the clinician and patient by explaining things more simply and clearly delineating all of the treatment options. Paskett noted that navigators are often trained with the PACE[4] technique, which helps patients learn how to talk to their health care clinicians. Oo added that at her facility, patient navigators not only explain cancer treatment and control, but also disease prevention and health promotion. Navigators also advocate for patients to ensure patient-centered care, planning, and goal setting.

---

[4] PACE is presenting information, asking questions, checking for understanding, and expressing concerns. See www.ncbi.nlm.nih.gov/pubmed/10664643 (accessed March 5, 2018).

Patient navigators also try to prevent or address insensitive or inappropriate communication about a patient's cancer, several workshop participants noted. William (Tony) Burns, cancer survivor, peer mentor, and advocate, noted that he received his cancer diagnosis over the phone by a stranger unfamiliar with him and his medical history rather than in person by his physician, who knew him well and about his history of human immunodeficiency virus (HIV), which contributed to his cancer. Cynthia Cantril, director of cancer support services and patient navigation at the Sutter Pacific Medical Foundation, relayed the story of a patient with breast cancer who was told of her diagnosis on a Friday by a radiologist, even though the patient had specified that she did not want to know her results until she had an appointment with the nurse navigator the following Wednesday—because her daughter was having a double mastectomy on Monday. Cantril said she also knew of a woman who got her breast cancer diagnosis while she was home alone with her toddler and 6-week-old twins. She said a diagnosis forever changes a person's life. How people hear about it sets the landscape for how they are going to perceive their care and trust their providers. She sought to explore patient preferences and change the way patients are informed of their cancer diagnosis.

Communication can also be inadequate when patients have treatment options that fall under the domain of different clinicians, said John Gardenier, a retired employee from the National Center for Health Statistics. Paskett agreed and noted that if a cancer patient is trying to make decisions about radiation therapy and surgery, the navigator will explain all of the different treatment options and help the patient assess which treatment decision is most appropriate for his or her personal situation. Freeman added that for patients diagnosed with prostate cancer, nurse navigators at the Ralph Lauren Center for Cancer Care in Harlem explain the meaning of an elevated level of prostate-specific antigen (PSA) and how a Gleason score[5] influences treatment options. "When we held hearings around the country we heard men who had prostate cancer who had never been told

[5] A Gleason score is "a system of grading prostate cancer tissue based on how it looks under a microscope. Gleason scores range from 2 to 10 and indicate how likely it is that a tumor will spread. A low Gleason score means the cancer tissue is similar to normal prostate tissue and the tumor is less likely to spread; a high Gleason score means the cancer tissue is very different from normal and the tumor is more likely to spread." See www.cancer.gov/publications/dictionaries/cancer-terms/def/gleason-score (accessed February 28, 2018).

anything except to cut it out, so it is a serious problem, particularly if you do not know there may be other options you could consider," Freeman said.

Patient navigators can also help foster communication between the patient and his or her family members and caregivers, said Alice Kerber, oncology and genetics clinical nurse specialist at Georgia Center for Oncology Research and Education (CORE).

Overcoming Health Care System Barriers

Several speakers and participants emphasized that a major role of the patient navigator is to fill gaps in the health care system. A review of the 2017 CoC survey of accredited cancer centers found that a fragmented medical system ranked highest among system barriers, said Miller. Lathan noted that at numerous points in the cancer care trajectory, patients can be lost to follow-up (Waldman et al., 2013) (see Figure 2).

"People who have less voice, people who are working every day, [and] people who are poor have a harder time continuing through this process," Lathan said. "Patients can feel lost in the system," Cantril added, and noted that at her health care system, the biggest issue for navigators is tracking patients throughout their trajectory of care with different clinicians and facilities.

Freeman stressed that patients often have to go to more than one facility for their cancer care and that patient navigation can virtually integrate a fragmented health care system for the individual patient. Such navigation can serve, for example, as the process that connects disconnected health care systems such as primary care and tertiary care sites, he said. Sometimes navigators close the gaps between clinicians by scheduling appointments for patients and ensuring preauthorization for the next steps of their care, Burbage noted. She also stressed how patient navigators can link patients and caregivers to resources within an institution and community, and ensure safe transitions of care across care settings.

Freeman gave the analogy of a relay race in which there are four runners who pass the baton to each other as they finish their portions of the race. The navigator makes sure the baton is passed to the next person in the health care trajectory, Freeman noted, such as from the community center where the cancer is detected to the radiologist or surgeon, who then must pass it to the medical oncologist. "The race is not over until you carry the baton across the finish line, and that is what patient navigation does. It is a team effort that aims toward resolution of some kind," he said. Nikolas Buescher,

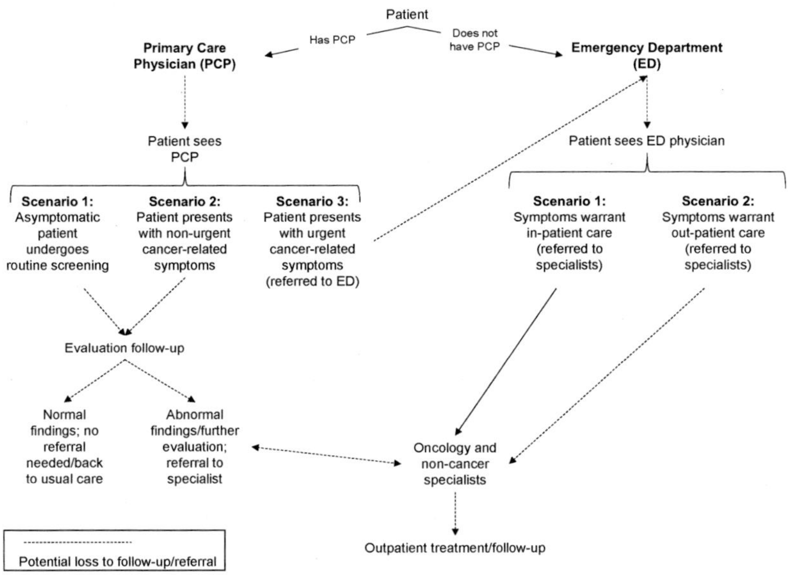

FIGURE 2 A cancer diagnosis and treatment pathway.
SOURCES: Lathan presentation, November 13, 2017; Reprinted from *Healthcare*, 1(3), Waldman, L. T., L. Svoboda, B. F. Young, G. A. Abel, S. Berlin, A. A. Elfiky, R. A. Freedman, M. Drews, L. Holland, and C. S. Lathan, A novel community-based delivery model to combat cancer disparities, 123–129, Copyright 2013, with permission from Elsevier.

executive director of Cancer Services at Penn Medicine/Lancaster General Health, noted that "every runner in that race has hundreds of batons that are currently going around the track at any given point in time, and the challenging part the navigator needs to figure out is which of those batons is most likely to drop, and if dropped, is going to break."

One of the gaps in cancer care can be transportation to a health care facility. According to Amy Bertrand, patient navigator at ACS, transportation was one of the bigger barriers for cancer patients at her health care facility, with many lacking cars or public transportation to take them to their treatment site. A review of the 2017 CoC accreditation survey results also found that transportation ranked as one of the most commonly cited barriers to care. At the University of Vermont Medical Center, patients often have to travel long distances for their care "so I assess right off, where are you coming from, and can you get here," Bertrand said. Valania added that many patients she helps with navigation are unable to afford public transportation to a cancer care facility.

Another important role of the navigator is to streamline care and facilitate timely treatment, several speakers noted. Paskett and her colleagues conducted a non-interventional, retrospective analysis of 1,786 Medicaid patients with late-stage breast cancer, and found a significant difference in mortality among those patients who experienced wait times of 2 months from the time they were diagnosed to the time they were first treated (McLaughlin et al., 2012). "So it is a lot more than just touchy feely stuff—navigation makes a difference in life and death," Paskett stressed. Linda Horn, cancer survivor and former chief executive officer of the Sutter Coast Hospital, noted that for cancer patients, "The hardest thing is when you sit in limbo. One of the most powerful things you can give back to your patients is to take something you have measured and improve it [like the time from positive pathology to first visit with the specialist], which gets the patients to the next step in their plan of care sooner." Raymond Osarogiagbon, hematologist and medical oncologist at the Baptist Cancer Center, agreed, noting that patients often say "Do not tell me I have a life-threatening illness and then make me wait." Cantril noted that when she first assessed her health care system, she discovered a substantial delay from the time a clinician was told the results of a patient's pathology report to the time of the patient's first medical oncology or surgical oncology consultation. This unnecessary delay was due to surgeons providing referrals to medical oncologists only postoperatively. She addressed this by recommending that primary care clinicians refer patients with positive pathology results from their biopsies to medical oncologists before they receive surgical treatment for their cancer. That way, a patient could meet with his or her surgeon and medical oncologist simultaneously, significantly shortening the time needed to devise a treatment plan.

Melissa Simon pointed out that patient navigators

> give us super important information by showing us all the gaps and bumps the patient is experiencing, such as which doctor is not following the guidelines, which clinic is not connected well enough to the lab to get results in an efficient way, and which imaging center is not calling their patients with their results. These are things for which we do not have the glasses with the right lenses to see and miss until the navigator shows us.

Oo noted that at her facility, patient navigators help patients access the services they need and help them get to their appointments. Horn emphasized the need for this because "when you are the cancer patient, there are times when you are tired, and physically and mentally struggling, and you are not always going to be able to be your strongest advocate." When Horn personally struggled with cancer, her nurse navigator had arranged her scans and clinician visits all in 1 day, knowing that it would take her 6 hours to make the round trip from her home to her cancer facility. The navigator also arranged for clinicians to give Horn second and third opinions about her care over the phone, and made sure those clinicians had access to her medical records. Horn quoted Freeman, who stated that "no patient should spend more time fighting the health care system than they do fighting their disease."

Building Trust and Providing Emotional Support

Several speakers suggested that another key role of the patient navigator is to help build patients' relationships with and trust of the medical system, and overcome their fears and anxieties. Providing emotional support for the patient is critical, Burbage said. Horn added that providing access to any needed psychosocial or spiritual care is also vital. Greg Simon noted that navigators can relieve patients' anxieties and fears by providing them with a vision of what is going to happen next and reassuring them that they will have the care they need. "I needed help from people who had been there before. That is you [patient navigators]," he said, and added, "We think of patient navigation too often as an extra, as an add-on, when in fact, it is the essence of the medical profession to do no harm. If you do not help people the moment they walk in the door, know everything that is going to happen, where, when, and how it is going to be, then you are harming them because that anxiety affects their health. It is bad enough to have cancer, but to have fear is worse."

He also said that emotional distress can interfere with patients' ability to adhere to their treatment plans. He described how the Eliza Corporation used an automated call system with artificial intelligence to contact people whose prescriptions were not filled to find out why they were not following their treatment plan.[6] He said many of the reasons given were not financial, but rather, for example, "the rest of my life is in shambles and I really did not worry about filling my prescription. People [with cancer] are fragile,

[6] See http://www.elizacorp.com/who-we-help/pharmacy-benefit-managers (accessed April 11, 2018).

and often depressed, or scared," Simon stressed, so they may need emotional support to enable adherence to their medical treatments.

Several participants pointed to the personalized support that navigators provide for patients and their caregivers. "We share with them face to face that there is somebody here that can help them navigate the different support services that they inevitably will need," Bertrand said. Freeman noted that along with the cancer treatments tailored to patients' particular genetic variants of cancer, there should also be personalized approaches to the patients' concerns.

Cantril noted that cancer patients often experience anxiety when they finish their treatment and that wellness programs and survivorship speaker series can help address that anxiety. Navigators, consequently, are still involved with patients after they complete their treatment at her facility. As Meneses pointed out, "One of the things we have learned is that you just cannot stop," and that navigators stay involved with patients during their survivorship care, and if the cancer continues to progress, during end-of-life care.

NAVIGATION THROUGHOUT THE CANCER CARE CONTINUUM

Both Freeman and Paskett emphasized that navigation services should be available throughout the cancer care continuum, from prevention and screening to diagnosis, treatment, and survivorship care (see Figure 3). "We need to be concerned about the patient moving to a resolution across the continuum of cancer care," Freeman said. Cantril noted that her facility aims to improve continuity of cancer care across the continuum by having the same nurse who educates patients about their chemotherapy also counsel them on their survivorship care plan.

Some participants also stressed the need for including patient navigation within end-of-life care. Stacy Fischer, associate professor at the University of Colorado School of Medicine, noted that some clinicians may avoid end-of-life discussions and that patient navigators can help patients ask their clinicians the right questions about care options. "We need to treat the prognosis and not just the diagnosis," Horn said. She suggested that patient navigators include a discussion about hospice care with their cancer patients. Valania stressed the need to improve the use of advance directives. When she has the opportunity, she discusses palliative medicine and hospice

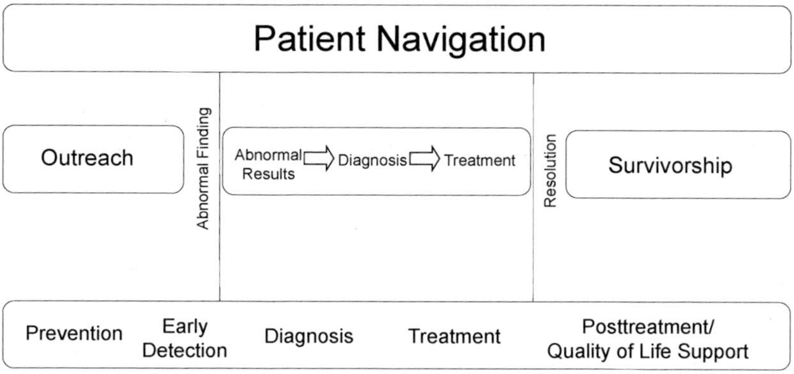

FIGURE 3 Patient navigation across the cancer care continuum.
SOURCES: Freeman presentation, November 13, 2017; adapted from Freeman, 2006.

referrals with the patients she navigates, but added that she needs clinician buy-in for those discussions to be useful.

EXAMPLES OF NAVIGATION SUCCESS STORIES

Several presenters gave anecdotal examples of how patient navigation has been helpful for them or for their patients. Paskett described a 51-year-old patient, who had a history of mental health issues, lacked transportation, had difficulty understanding instructions, worked in a blue-collar job, and lived alone. When he presented to his primary care clinician with rectal bleeding and pain, his clinician recommended a colonoscopy as soon as possible. He had a navigator, who worked with him for months. This navigator rescheduled his colonoscopy three times, coached him on how to take the prep treatment, and drove him to and from the hospital because he had nobody else to take him for the procedure. She helped him determine that he could use a vacation day for his colonoscopy and scheduled it on Monday so he could spend Sunday at home doing his prep treatment. The colonoscopy revealed a 5-centimeter polyp. "The navigator prevented a cancer in this gentleman by not letting him be lost to follow-up and by encouraging him and teaching him how to be his own navigator," Paskett said.

Tony Burns and his sister, Doris Burns, who both had cancer and lived in an impoverished neighborhood, stressed the importance of their patient navigators and a navigation system at the facility where they were treated. "I could not have done this alone and I thank God that I did not have to—it was the doctors, the care navigators, the administrative staff, nurses, and the system that helped me," Tony Burns said. Doris Burns added, "Without the cancer navigation system being in place, neither I nor my brother Tony would have been able to obtain the care, the treatment, or the support that we received. My recommendation for those present today is that you do everything within your power to keep these systems and services in place." Tony Burns said, "Sometimes life gets crazy when you are marginalized. But when you have folks that give you a place and give you an ear, it helps lift you up. And then it helps lift the community up."

Aditi Narayan, senior manager of patient support and research at the LIVESTRONG Foundation, told the story of a cancer survivor who contacted LIVESTRONG's patient navigation program after being diagnosed with brain cancer. He wanted to know how to seek a second opinion because the first clinician he saw told him he would never be able to run again—and he was a marathon runner. A navigator helped him learn how to express his personal goals to his clinicians so he could make decisions and act as part of the team. He made it clear to them that it was a high priority for him to run in a qualifying marathon before his treatment started, which enabled him to run in the subsequent Boston Marathon after his treatment.

WHO SHOULD RECEIVE NAVIGATION SERVICES?

A number of workshop participants asked which patients should receive navigation services, with some presenters suggesting all patients can benefit from such services, while others, recognizing the limited and variable resources available to support navigation in some health care systems, suggested navigation be limited to those patients who need it most. Freeman noted that "anyone with cancer would benefit from some extra help, even if you are a billionaire, but in the real world we probably cannot pay for navigating everybody." He suggested patient navigation be a targeted intervention for patients at high risk for delays in cancer care, because delays are linked to poorer outcomes. Patients at risk would include those with low economic status, those with limited education or health literacy, and those lacking insurance, he said. Buescher advocated for finding patients who need navigation support, rather than relying on them to self-identify. "We are trying to distinguish between being reactive firefighters to now being a little more of a proactive smoke detector and trying to identify in advance who is most likely to need navigation services," he said.

Bertrand argued that every cancer patient needs access to navigation, although not all patients require face-to-face navigation. She noted that informational handouts can be given to patients when they are first seen for their cancer care. These handouts can provide information on how to contact patient navigators when needed. "So if somebody does not necessarily need me right off, I know that they are likely to pop up because I planted a seed. I have had either an opportunity to meet them, or they have information along their journey to be able to have access to a navigator," Bertrand said.

Valania said her facility does not have enough resources to provide navigation for all cancer patients, so instead patients are prioritized by need. "Right now I am really just putting out the fires," she said, and stressed that better assessments are needed to identify which patients need navigation services the most. She noted that distress screening tools are often unreliable because of their subjectivity, adding, "Do not just ask patients if they are distressed, but rather uncover what is happening to them that is making them feel distressed. If your patient needs a shorter walk from the car to the office, let's get him a wheelchair. They do not need a social worker. There are just not enough support services right now."

A number of workshop participants noted common red flags for patients needing cancer care navigation include people at risk of being lost to follow-up and those with concurrent illnesses. Many patients have more than one red flag signaling the need for patient navigation. In an analysis of 1,995 and 1,194 patients with breast and cervical abnormalities, respectively, Paskett and colleagues found that patients most likely to have barriers to care were those who were low income, unemployed, less educated, renters, not married, or had two or more dependents (Katz et al., 2014). Another study of 424 patients found that patients most likely to report a barrier to receiving care were those who were people of color, less educated, unemployed, retired, low income, or uninsured, and those with other illnesses (Krok-Schoen et al., 2015). Concurring with those findings, Paskett reported on another study, with 3,777 participants, that found that those benefitting the most from navigation were patients who were poorer, sicker, and unemployed (Rodday et al., 2015).

A few workshop participants stressed that high-acuity patients (those with complex care needs) also are more likely to benefit from patient navigation. Osarogiagbon noted that lung cancer is a high-acuity cancer because it requires an invasive procedure for diagnosis, and the clinicians responsible for the various diagnostic, staging, and treatment modalities tend to be different types of specialists with different practices that are traditionally not well integrated. The end result is a fragmented system for delivering care to lung cancer patients. These patients also tend to be older and are more likely to smoke, and thus have several tobacco-related concurrent conditions that can further complicate the delivery of complex care.

Burbage noted that at her facility, navigators use an acuity scale that not only takes into account socioeconomic factors (e.g., whether patients have sufficient insurance and housing, and can afford transportation), but also the different modalities of treatment that may be recommended, concurrent illnesses (including psychiatric and substance use disorders), and English proficiency and health literacy. An acuity rating is also based on whether patients have a support system and whether they are caregivers for others, such as children or elderly parents. Burbage added that it is challenging to balance the volume and acuity of patients with the limited resources for navigation, and suggested perhaps having group visits for people at high risk for cancer or the survivorship population, and saving individual visits for those who need it the most.

WHO NAVIGATES?

Several workshop participants reported on the different types of patient navigators, from lay or peer navigators to professionals, such as nurses and social workers, and debated which types were most appropriate. Some pointed out, however, that the answer to this question depends in part on the circumstances of the patient population needing navigation services.

Freeman stressed that the required level of skills varies. He noted that at Harlem Hospital, lay navigators handle issues such as insurance, tracking patients through the health care system, alleviating fear, etc. "If you are dealing with disparities, the non-clinical navigator can have the power to solve most of these issues and can call in specialists, such as a social worker, when those problems are severe," Freeman said. Once a patient has a cancer diagnosis, nurses play a bigger role, but the lay navigator continues to stay with the patients and makes sure they understand what the nurses and physicians are saying, he added. He noted that a lack of insurance or understanding of where to go for cancer screening are key factors that cause late diagnosis and are best addressed by lay navigators, while professional navigators with medical expertise can handle the clinical issues. "A team of lay and nurse and other professional navigators should work together, particularly at the point of a cancer diagnosis," Freeman said. Mandi Pratt-Chapman, associate center director of patient-centered initiatives and health equity at the George Washington University Cancer Center, agreed that "teams of navigators are most ideal but are not always possible in a resource-constrained environment, but I am a big fan of multidisciplinary teamwork, even within the navigation team."

Paskett responded by noting there are many different models of navigation, and at her institution all patient navigators are lay navigators who are coordinated by a social worker because "you have to have a conductor for the symphony." The lay navigators provide emotional counseling, and consult with a nurse when needed. "The nurses and whole clinical team cannot get through a day without the lay navigator. It is a symbiotic relationship," Paskett said.

Burbage noted that patient navigators are also sometimes referred to as community health workers, patient managers, or case coordinators, among a dozen other titles she has discovered in the literature. She reported that an oncology nurse navigator is defined as a registered nurse with oncology-specific clinical knowledge who offers individual assistance to patients, families, and caregivers to help overcome health care system barriers using the nursing process (ONS, 2017). Oncology nurse navigators also provide education and resources to facilitate informed decision making throughout the cancer continuum. By contrast, a lay navigator is defined as a trained non-professional or volunteer who provides individualized assistance to patients, families, and caregivers to help overcome health care system barriers, and facilitates timely access to quality health and psychosocial care (ONS, 2017).

Oncology nurse navigators often have a bachelor of science degree in nursing and are generally certified in oncology, whereas lay navigators tend to be volunteers or are supported with grant funds, may have a history of a cancer diagnosis, and often work in specific areas of the community where they live and are trusted, such as community health centers and houses of worship, according to Burbage. She noted that the most robust navigation programs have a combination of both nurse and lay navigators who work closely together. Oncology social workers can also function as patient navigators. Social worker navigators perform initial and ongoing psychosocial assessments, assist patients and caregivers with social care needs, and link patients and caregivers to community resources. Social workers usually have a master of social work degree, and may be certified in oncology (ONS, 2017).

George Weiner, professor and director of the Holden Comprehensive

Cancer Center at The University of Iowa, asked when to employ a nurse navigator versus a lay navigator. Burbage responded that her facility generally relies on nurse navigators to provide education, but patients are made aware that if they would like to speak with someone, lay navigators are available. She added that there is close communication between the lay and nurse navigators responsible for the same patient. For example, the lay navigator may let the nurse navigator know that the patient is still confused about the diagnosis or treatment and needs a better explanation.

Pratt-Chapman stressed that although both lay and nurse navigators have some of the same roles and skill sets, some responsibilities are best addressed by nurse navigators. These responsibilities include providing and reinforcing education to patients, families, and caregivers regarding diagnosis, treatment options, management of side effects, posttreatment care, and survivorship (ONS, 2017).

As a peer navigator for people living with HIV, Tony Burns added that there is a value to having been through what the patient is about to experience that enables the navigator to serve as a useful bridge between the patient and the clinician. He said he accompanies patients to their clinic visits and "breaks down what [clinicians] say into layman terms."

Paskett noted that her institution tries to engage lay navigators from the same communities as their patients. For example, it hires and trains Somali, African American, and Appalachian lay navigators. However, Burns noted,

> We really are a village, but sometimes we get tribal. It's good to know when I'm looking at someone who doesn't share my ethnicity that I can say it like I feel it. One of the blessings I've had is to be able to look at a doctor that is a white man or white woman and see that they care something about me as a human being. That has meant the world for me and has helped to inspire me to be engaged in my care.

Kerber noted that she often wondered, while working as a nurse in the hospital, "why patients spill their guts to the housekeepers," and not the medical staff. She suspects that is because a nurse "has a sharp object in her hand, but the housekeepers are the ones that are doing normal stuff. Sometimes you just want to talk to somebody who is doing normal stuff, someone you can relate to, whether it is in terms of what you do, your financial capabilities, or other traits." Meneses pointed out that because the navigators in the Patient Care Connect Program (PCCP) all live in the local community in which the patients reside, they have a strong understanding of the health disparities that need to be addressed. Kerber added that "Some of our best navigators are the patients themselves and their families, who help us determine what we need to do."

EVIDENCE ON PATIENT NAVIGATION

A number of workshop participants reviewed the evidence gathered to date on the benefits of patient navigation in oncology. Paskett said she and her colleagues (including Battaglia and Melissa Simon) conducted a randomized, multisite study of more than 10,000 patients with cervical, breast, and colorectal cancer, most of whom were people of color and were publicly insured or uninsured (Freund et al., 2014). This PNRP study found that navigation significantly decreased the amount of time between when an abnormality was first detected and when a patient was given a cancer diagnosis. This study also found that navigation significantly reduced the time between diagnosis and the start of treatment.

A secondary analysis of this study found that navigation eliminated disparities in cancer outcomes due to differences in income, employment status, and presence of concurrent diseases (Rodday et al., 2015). "This study showed that in a large diverse population, patient navigation reduced delays to receiving follow-up care for cancer abnormalities, reduced delays in starting cancer treatment, and reduced the number of patients lost to follow-up by about 20 percent. The study also showed that patient navigation helped patients most in need and at risk for delays in treatment," Paskett stressed.

Paskett also reported that her review of 29 studies on patient navigation conducted between 2010 and 2015 (mostly for patients with breast cancer, but also patients with cervical, colorectal, and lung cancer) found that the majority showed patient navigation to be effective in increasing screening rates and reducing time to diagnosis and treatment, as well as improving care plan adherence, quality of life, patient knowledge, and communication with clinicians (Krok-Schoen et al., 2016). More recently, one randomized, controlled clinical trial found that patient navigation increased rates of colorectal cancer screening compared with usual care in a vulnerable population (Reuland et al., 2017), and an observational study found that patient navigation reduced costs, emergency room visits, hospitalizations, and intensive care unit admissions compared with controls in a Medicare population (Rocque et al., 2017). This resulted in an estimated savings of $19 million in health care costs, Paskett reported, with a return on investment of 1 to 10 (Rocque et al., 2017), Meneses noted. Another observational study[7] reported by Burbage found that the implementation of a patient navigation program at a breast center was followed by substantially reduced average time from an abnormal finding to a breast biopsy result. Emergency room visits also fell to nearly half of what they were prior to program implementation. Hospital admission and readmission rates also declined after the program was implemented.

Kris Blackley, director of patient navigation at the Levine Cancer Institute, described a study of patients at her facility that showed that the patients who did not receive navigation services were 52 percent more likely to have unplanned hospital readmissions within 30 days, compared with patients who had these services (Kowalkowski et al., 2016a). In a retrospective cohort study of approximately 2,300 patients with poor prognosis (as defined by the ACS), Blackley and colleagues found a significant survival benefit for patients who had received navigation services compared with those who had not (Kowalkowski et al., 2016b). The greatest survival advantage was seen in patients who were African American, who were insured by Medicaid, or who had lung or pancreatic cancer, said Blackley.

Lori Hoffman Hōgg, national oncology clinical advisor at the Department of Veterans Affairs, said a study demonstrated that using nurse navigation improved the early detection of lung cancer at a hospital in the Connecticut Veterans Affairs Healthcare System. Following implementation of patient navigation, the percentage of patients with non-small-cell lung cancer diagnosed at Stage I or II increased from 33 percent in 2006 to 53 percent in 2011, and the average time from first suspicion of cancer to start of treatment decreased from 136 days in 2003 to 55 days in 2010 (Hunnibell et al., 2012). Pratt-Chapman added that a study done at The University of Alabama at Birmingham found reductions in unplanned hospital admissions and emergency room visits, with a mean savings of $781.29 per quarter per patient after instituting a comprehensive navigation process, including advance directive counseling for high-risk patients and geriatric patients (Rocque et al., 2017).

Cantril reported on studies showing that a lack of nurse navigation resulted in more days of treatment interruption (Krebs et al., 2013), longer times to diagnostic resolution (Basu et al., 2013), an increase in time to first clinician visit/treatment (Gordils-Perez, 2017), an increased length of time between procedures (Harding and McCrone, 2013), and more lost or missing test results (Harding and McCrone, 2013). A lack of nurse navigation

[7] Unpublished internal data.

was also linked to patients' loss of trust in health care teams, higher levels of patient anxiety and distress, and lower levels of patient satisfaction, as well as dissatisfaction with information and impressions of having a dehumanizing experience (Harding and McCrone, 2013).

"We have enough evidence to say that patient navigation works in most of the cancer care continuum, in many populations, and for several outcomes," Paskett said.

EXAMPLES OF RESEARCH NEEDS

Paskett pointed out several gaps in the evidence on patient navigation. Few studies have been conducted in the posttreatment setting, she noted, and only a limited number were conducted in the treatment setting. Virtually no studies have been reported that assess how navigation affects palliative care. "These are big holes to fill," she stressed. In addition, researchers need to assess the effects of navigation in a wider spectrum of cancers. Most navigation studies have focused on patients with breast cancer. Paskett also suggested studies with more innovative designs in real-world settings, noting that randomized controlled trials, although the gold standard, are limited by funding constraints. Implementation science studies might offer some solutions, she added (see Box 3).

Paskett also suggested expanding the metrics assessed in navigation studies to include the number of missed appointments, as well as patient satisfaction with care, mortality, costs, and return on investments. Osarogiagbon also stressed that measuring timeliness of care is a critical benchmark for patients and their caregivers, and that it can serve as a surrogate for their satisfaction with their care. But he cautioned that in one of his studies, timeliness of care correlated with a lack of necessary intermediary steps that should have been taken with lung cancer patients, resulting in inappropriate staging and treatment (Faris et al., 2015). "So hurrying up may not necessarily be as valuable as you might think for a complex disease such as lung cancer. We have to understand our benchmarks and what they are measuring," Osarogiagbon said.

Financial metrics are especially important, Paskett noted, for making the business case for patient navigation that hopefully will garner the funding to make it a more sustainable enterprise. Buescher and Cantril agreed, suggesting that studies measure the return on investment in navigation at the local level, incorporating information that is useful for "frontline managers" to devise strategies for their hospitals. "When a hospital administrator says to

BOX 3
Translating Research into Practice

Tracy Battaglia, associate professor of medicine and epidemiology at the Boston University School of Medicine, reported on a large, multisite pragmatic clinical trial called Translating Research Into Practice (TRIP),[a] which is supported by a grant from the National Center for Advancing Translational Sciences. This innovative dissemination and implementation science study aims to improve the delivery of timely, high-quality breast cancer care for vulnerable patients in Boston through a coordinated care delivery model. This model includes a patient navigator network that coordinates the efforts of all patient navigators across health care systems, a registry or tracking system to identify patients most at risk for delays in care that is sharable across health systems, and a platform to both screen for and address barriers related to the social determinants of health in low-income populations.

Clinical partners in TRIP include six of the health care systems in Boston that care for more than 90 percent of the at-risk populations, said Battaglia. Other community partners include the Boston Breast Cancer Equity Coalition and the Boston Patient Navigator Network. Patients are eligible for the program if they have a vulnerable risk factor, such as having public health insurance or not speaking English. The study uses a pragmatic stepped-wedge hybrid effectiveness design, an innovative research method to collect data in real-world clinical settings, with the goal of enrolling approximately 1,200 women.

The ultimate goal of TRIP is to eliminate care delivery disparities in this breast cancer population, and to serve as a model for other locations and other diseases, said Battaglia. The researchers are using frameworks for dissemination and implementation science so that their model can be applied to other health care systems and other diseases if they obtain positive results.

---

[a] See http://grantome.com/grant/NIH/U01-TR002070-01 (accessed March 6, 2018).
SOURCE: Battaglia presentation, November 13, 2017.

me, 'How we can afford navigators?' my response is 'How can we not afford navigators?'" Cantril said. Christine Evans, director of nursing at OncoNav, added that researchers and institutions should consider capturing data on how patient navigation affects out-migration of patients to another hospital or clinic. Cantril responded that sometimes newly diagnosed patients she encounters at her facility are less likely to seek a second opinion at another facility once they understand that she can arrange multidisciplinary care for them. Cantril also suggested that if her facility improves care through a patient navigation program, that could foster greater in-migration to a facility. "We don't capture [data on] how many new patients are coming to us because we are doing a good job," Cantril stressed. Freeman quoted Albert Einstein, who said, "Not everything that counts can be counted, and not everything that can be counted counts." Freeman stressed, "We have to be sure we are counting the things that really count. We might be counting a lot of things that look good scientifically, but maybe they are not the right things that count when doing patient navigation."

REAL-WORLD MODELS OF PATIENT NAVIGATION

A number of workshop participants also described patient navigation real-world models, including

- Christiana Care Health System Navigation Program
- Women's Wellness Connection Navigation Program
- American Cancer Society Patient Navigation Program
- Cancer Patient Navigators of Georgia
- LIVESTRONG Cancer Navigation Program
- Wayfinder Patient Navigation Program
- DuPage Patient Navigation Collaborative
- Dana-Farber Cancer Institute Patient Navigation Pilot
- Massachusetts General Hospital Patient Navigation Programs
- Apoyo con Cariño Palliative Care Program
- Patient Care Connect Program
- Sutter Health Patient Navigation Program
- Blue Distinction® Cancer Care Program
- Geisinger Oncology Navigator Program

Christiana Care Health System Navigation Program

Burbage reported on the patient navigation services at the Christiana Care Health System, a 1,100-bed nonprofit teaching institution in Newark, Delaware. First implemented in 1999 to coincide with the opening of a breast center, this navigation program was based on input from patients about what had helped them after they were diagnosed with cancer. The navigation program expanded to include patients diagnosed with other types of cancer by 2001, and expanded again in 2010 to include navigation services for cancer survivorship care. By 2017, the navigation program included a supportive and palliative care component.

Disease-specific oncology nurse navigators staff the program, including in-patient nurse navigators who help improve the discharge planning process. In addition, the program has social workers and lay navigators who work in their community health and outreach program. Burbage serves as the leader and coordinator for all of the navigators, whose caseloads vary between 50 and 100 patients at various points along the cancer care continuum.

The majority of the lay navigators are either supported by grants, such as those from the Avon Foundation for Women or Susan G. Komen, or state funding resources. These lay navigators are either bilingual, in Spanish and English or Mandarin and English, or are African American. Some lay navigators also focus on prevention and specialize in screening for breast, cervical, colorectal, prostate, and lung cancers.

Burbage reported that since the implementation of the patient navigation program, the breast biopsy turnaround time (from an abnormal finding to biopsy result) has decreased from 18 days to 5 days. They also compared emergency room visits, hospital admissions, and readmissions of patients with and without navigation support. Among patients without navigation services, 58 percent (28/48) had emergency room visits, 33 percent were admitted to the hospital, and 31 percent of those patients were readmitted within 30 days. Among patients with navigation support, 31 percent (14/45) had emergency room visits, 26 percent were admitted to the hospital, and only 15 percent of those were readmitted within 30 days.

Women's Wellness Connection Navigation Program

Kris McCracken, program coordinator of the Women's Wellness Connection (WWC) at the Colorado Department of Public Health and Environment, reported on the patient navigation strategy deployed by WWC, a breast and cervical cancer screening program in Colorado that is funded by the Centers for Disease Control and Prevention and encompasses more than 130 clinics. The goal of WWC is to reduce breast and cervical cancer morbidity, mortality, and disparities by providing, promoting, and ensuring quality breast and cervical cancer screening for underserved women in Colorado, and by connecting them to the necessary resources. In addition to reimbursing the clinics in its network for providing breast and cervical cancer screening, diagnostic testing, and referrals to treatment for uninsured or underinsured women, WWC also reimburses them for navigation services to guide the women through the screening and follow-up process.

McCracken said that patient navigation has been a part of WWC's clinical services for many years, but after the implementation of the ACA, WWC added a patient navigation program for low-income, insured women called the Care Coordination Grant Program.[8] "We started this new patient navigation program because we know that even though they have adequate health insurance to pay for cancer screening, many women still face substantial barriers to obtaining those screenings, such as geographic isolation or limited health literacy," she said.

The program was instituted in 26 health organizations and involves assessment and resolution of barriers to completion of screening, diagnostic, and treatment services. It requires a minimum of two contacts with each client over the course of the screening and diagnostic cycle. Since the expanded patient navigation program was implemented, nearly 11,000 insured women have received navigation services that helped them complete breast and cervical cancer screenings, diagnostic testing, and referrals to treatment. Eighty-three cases of breast cancer and 61 cases of cervical cancer were diagnosed in this population. "That's almost 150 women who we likely helped by finding their cancer earlier," McCracken stressed.

American Cancer Society Patient Navigation Program

Bertrand reported on the ACS Patient Navigation Program, which consists of more than 100 patient navigators who usually work in large cancer centers that are certified by the CoC, or systems that provide care to large populations with a significant percentage of medically underserved individuals. Trained navigators work with patients and caregivers from the time

[8] See www.colorado.gov/pacific/cancerplan/program-manual (accessed March 8, 2018).

of diagnosis and throughout treatment to ensure they have understandable and up-to-date information about their cancer. ACS navigators also provide practical assistance for patients and their caregivers, such as linking them to transportation, lodging, financial, and other needed resources. Patient navigator training and support is a shared responsibility of the ACS and the host health care facility. To ensure continuous program quality improvement, evaluation, monitoring, and tracking are key components to the success of the program, she said.

Cancer Patient Navigators of Georgia

Kerber reported on the Cancer Patient Navigators of Georgia (CPNG), a statewide virtual organization of patient navigators with the mission of connecting, educating, and sharing best practices among patient navigators in Georgia to reduce barriers to care and increase services related to cancer. Participants in the organization include nurses, lay navigators, physicians, social workers, and public health workers.

CPNG has a website,[9] provides a newsletter for its nearly 400 members, and holds an annual conference at which participants can receive training on topics such as metrics and integrative therapies, share best practices, and network. CPNG receives its support from the Georgia CORE and the Georgia Society of Clinical Oncology, and participates in a variety of working groups within the Georgia Comprehensive Cancer Control Plan.

LIVESTRONG Cancer Navigation Program

Narayan reported on the LIVESTRONG Cancer Navigation program, which was designed to be a central hub of support for cancer survivors and their family and friends. The program, which addresses physical, emotional, and practical concerns in partnership with best-in-class organizations, was designed to complement what is already offered in a clinical setting. The program provides referrals to other organizations when it cannot directly address the issue, such as emotional counseling and peer support, with the goal of "reducing the burden on cancer survivors by being their champion and cheerleader," said Narayan.

After patients contact the program by phone or online, navigators complete a detailed needs assessment that tries to identify "the root cause of each

[9] See http://www.gacancerpatientnavigators.org (accessed March 8, 2018).

survivor's pain points because there is typically more than one thing that is contributing to their distress," Narayan said. The navigator will then help the patients overcome their challenges in a timely manner. The program adopted the National Comprehensive Cancer Network distress thermometer[10] and the comprehensive score for financial toxicity[11] to better assess their clients' needs. Navigators also try to help survivors feel empowered to ask questions of their clinicians and express their personal goals for care.

In 2016, the program served nearly 10,000 individuals and helped approximately 2,600 clients save more than $11 million with debt relief and by supporting the cost of living and costs associated with fertility preservation, said Narayan. LIVESTRONG conducted a study of 761 cancer survivors who used its navigation program between March 2011 and October 2012 and found that the mean distress score significantly decreased and mean self-efficacy scores increased (Treiman et al., 2015). Since that study, however, Narayan said LIVESTRONG has stopped providing direct counseling services in its navigation program, although it does make referrals and helps facilitate direct connections to counseling.

Wayfinder Patient Navigation Program

Paskett reported on the Wayfinder patient navigation program, which is funded by multiple sources, including The Ohio State University, Susan G. Komen, a breast clinic, a family practice clinic, a gastroenterology clinic, and a gynecology clinic. Paskett said the need for patient navigation at the Breast Center of The Ohio State University Comprehensive Cancer Center is so great that navigators there only work with Medicaid and minority patients. "We don't have enough staff to meet the need," Paskett said.

The goals of Wayfinder are to increase use of preventive services among the Medicaid population, and to reduce no-shows and cancellations. Paskett said initial, unpublished data from the first 6 months of the program showed that no-show rates were reduced by 40 percent for colposcopy, and by 80 percent for endoscopy. The 6-month data also showed that the number of Medicaid patients overdue for a mammogram was cut in half,

[10] See https://www.nccn.org/patients/resources/life_with_cancer/pdf/nccn_distress_thermometer.pdf (accessed February 27, 2018).

[11] See http://onlinelibrary.wiley.com/doi/10.1002/cncr.28814/full (accessed March 8, 2018) and https://www.ncbi.nlm.nih.gov/pmc/articles/PMC5298039 (accessed March 8, 2018).

for a colon cancer screen was decreased by nearly one-third, and for cervical cancer screening was reduced by about one-fifth.

DuPage Patient Navigation Collaborative

Melissa Simon reported on the DuPage Patient Navigation Collaborative (DPNC) in DuPage County, Illinois. This county has about 1 million people, including a number of Mexican immigrants who are not proficient in English, she said. DuPage also lacks public transportation aligned with health and human services, which increases the need for patient navigation. DPNC provides navigation services aimed at improving breast and cervical cancer screening and treatment for women. The program engages community health workers or patient navigators through a freestanding community organization called Access DuPage. These navigators have no allegiance to a particular health care system, hospital, or clinic, and can leverage every community health and human service across the entire county.

A study of the navigation collaborative found that compared with English-speaking patients, Spanish-speaking patients had lower incomes, health literacy, and patient activation, and were more distrustful of the health system (Samaras et al., 2014). Despite these challenges, the collaborative appeared to mitigate the health disparities among these patients. For example, there were no differences in the likelihood of follow-up delays of greater than 60 days by language, and patients entering the study with higher health care system distrust had a lower likelihood of delayed follow-up time after abnormal cervical screening. The study also found that DPNC strengthened community partnerships and enhanced referral processes, communications, and service delivery among clinical teams (Samaras et al., 2014). "It didn't just help individual patients; it helped the community organizations and the health and human services organizations connect to each other at a county level," Simon said.

Dana-Farber Cancer Institute Patient Navigation Pilot

Lathan reported on the Dana-Farber Cancer Institute patient navigation pilot program, whose mission is to create more streamlined access to a cancer center and greater access to clinical trials for newly diagnosed patients, and to counter health disparities. Built around a nurse navigator, this program is funded by a philanthropic grant and is embedded in the primary care setting of a federally qualified community health center that serves mostly African Americans and immigrants from the Dominican Republic. The primary care clinicians refer any patient with a health issue that might be oncology related to the nurse navigator. Such issues are broadly defined, according to Lathan, and include a low white blood cell count and unexplained weight loss, for example. A medical oncologist then works with the nurse navigator to triage referred patients to care at a community cancer clinic or at the Dana-Farber Cancer Institute.

At the community cancer clinic, oncologists have formal and informal consultations with the primary care clinicians, and provide educational sessions for clinicians. Oncologists also consult with individual patients at the clinic, and provide community-level education sessions for patients. Lathan stressed that the oncologists function as generalists when consulting with primary care clinicians. "When I went to the clinic, I wasn't acting as a lung cancer doctor. I was seeing whatever issues came up," Lathan said. He stressed that "the key is our nurse navigator," an oncology nurse who is fluent in five languages. The pilot program also integrates lung cancer screening, tobacco cessation treatment, and genetic testing and counseling.

Lathan said that the program was structured to "keep as much in the community health center as possible," with none of the revenue from the oncology consults going to the Dana-Farber Cancer Institute. "It is all about staying and helping the individual Federally Qualified Health Center,"[12] Lathan said. However, some patients with cancer are referred to the Dana-Farber Cancer Institute for biopsies, imaging, chemotherapy, and palliative care.

Since the initiation of the patient navigation pilot program in January 2012, there have been 736 patient visits: 431 new patients and 305 follow-up visits, said Lathan. Forty-two percent of the patients seen had a hematologic or oncologic issue. Nearly 60 percent of patients continued to receive care at the community health center, while about 20 percent were referred to Dana-Farber Cancer Institute or Brigham and Women's Hospital. Fifteen percent of all patients with a cancer diagnosis entered a clinical trial (nearly 25 percent of patients in active treatment).

---

[12] Federally Qualified Health Centers "are community-based health care providers that receive funds from the Health Resources and Services Administration Health Center Program to provide primary care services in underserved areas. They must meet a stringent set of requirements, including providing care on a sliding fee scale based on ability to pay and operating under a governing board that includes patients." See https://www.hrsa.gov/opa/eligibility-and-registration/health-centers/fqhc/index.html (accessed April 11, 2018).

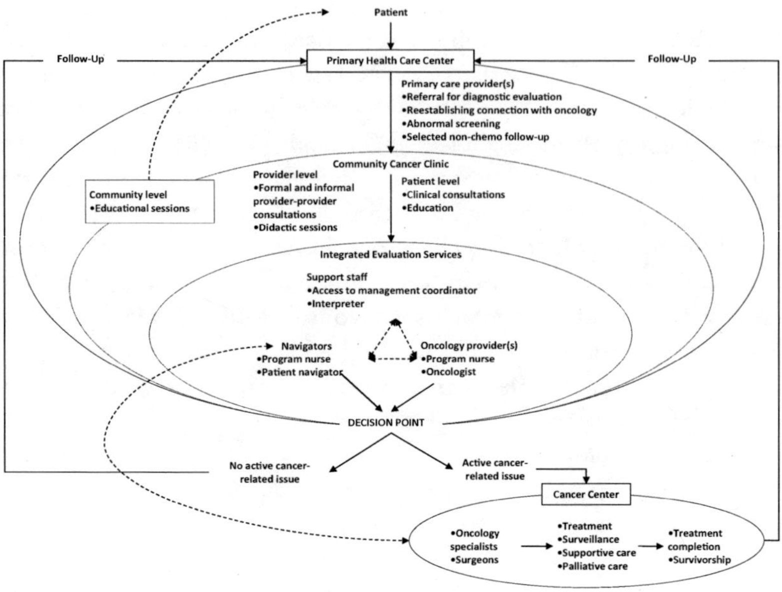

FIGURE 4 Conceptual model for a clinical outreach program.
SOURCES: Lathan presentation, November 13, 2017; Reprinted from *Healthcare*, 1(3), Waldman, L. T., L. Svoboda, B. F. Young, G. A. Abel, S. Berlin, A. A. Elfiky, R. A. Freedman, M. Drews, L. Holland, and C. S. Lathan, A novel community-based delivery model to combat cancer disparities, 123–129, Copyright 2013, with permission from Elsevier.

Prior to program implementation, the median time for clinical resolution after first reporting potential oncology-related symptoms was 19 days. Five years into the program, the median time to clinical resolution of patient visits was reduced to 12.5 days.

Lathan noted the Dana-Farber Cancer Institute pilot program model enables the integration of prevention programs, increases the flow of patients to the cancer center, strengthens the bonds in the community, and can be used in many different care settings and clinics (see Figure 4).

Massachusetts General Hospital Patient Navigation Programs

Oo reported on MGH Chelsea HealthCare Center's programs and strategies designed to assist refugees and immigrants from Africa, Central America, the Middle East, and Nepal. Oo said much of the patient population served by the Chelsea clinic has a history of trauma, extreme poverty, isolation, low literacy, and language barriers.

The clinic uses 45 community health workers from 25 countries who speak 21 languages. These health workers are funded by a number of sources, including foundations, grateful patients, and the Massachusetts Department of Public Health. "We created positions over time, showed them to be effective, and then the hospital supported them with their dollars," Oo said. The program does not focus on cancer, but rather on managing chronic diseases, navigating access to hospital services and community resources, and supporting adherence to treatment plans. The health workers help patients with all of their medical appointments, including cancer screenings. The community health workers are paired to patients with similar cultural backgrounds (i.e., if a patient is from Somalia, they are matched to a Somali health worker).

The responsibilities of community health workers include cultural mediation; providing culturally appropriate education on health promotion, disease prevention, treatment, and control; coordinating care; and managing cases. These navigators also help patients find their way in the health system, provide social support advocacy, and coach patients with the aim of building skills and self-efficacy, so patients can confidently care for their own health. Health workers also do outreach to patients who are difficult to engage, and act as a bridge between patient and clinician to ensure patient-centered care and planning that conforms to the patient's wishes and goals. "A lot of times health workers bridge the disconnect between where the patient is and where the provider is and advocate for the patient because the patient's voice is important," Oo stressed. She noted that many patients are refugees from war-torn countries or have experienced domestic violence. "So making sure the patient has a voice is critical. As soon as we start to take away the patients' voice we are retraumatizing them, even if we think it is in their best interest," Oo said. "We may think this colonoscopy is what they need to do now, but it is their decision," she noted.

Although the Chelsea health workers may have specialties, there is cross-training with clear systems of protocols and detailed manuals, so they each can provide navigation services for cancer care. "If they are making an early childhood home visit, and find their patient's [mother] is dealing with an overdue mammogram screening, they put on the navigator hat and address that," Oo said.

Since 2001, the Chelsea clinic has provided navigation services to more than 16,000 people receiving breast, cervical, or colorectal cancer screening and follow-up care, said Oo. In the clinic's Avon Breast Care Program, 92 percent of patients arrived for their first follow-up appointment within 60 days or less of being informed of an abnormal finding, said Oo. Navigators in the program arranged what Oo called "one-stop shopping," in which appointments with different clinicians could all be made on the same day at the same health care facility with a translator provided, if needed. This program has expanded to serve residents in the North Shore of Boston, in addition to Chelsea.

After developing a breast cancer screening program for Latinas, Oo said that MGH wanted to develop one for refugee women, particularly Arabic-speaking women from Africa or the Middle East. Recruiting, retaining, and financially supporting navigators for each group has been a major challenge, Oo said, so MGH also trained medical interpreters to provide navigation services for these populations. Culturally sensitive patient materials were provided to patients after navigators spoke to them about their cancer beliefs (Percac-Lima et al., 2013). For example, some materials stressed that women needed to attend cancer screening appointments so they could continue to take care of their relatives. Recognizing that some Somali patients could not read, the educational materials they created for these patients had many diagrams and pictures. "Each group was very different and we did whatever was appropriate in terms of encouraging women to get their screenings done," Oo said. This effort appeared to help reduce disparities in breast cancer screening rates between the refugee populations and those who spoke English or Spanish (Percac-Lima et al., 2013), Oo reported, although screening rates in the refugee populations are still below that of the others in Chelsea.

In 2005, an analysis found large disparities in colorectal cancer screening rates between whites and Latinos (61 percent versus 41 percent) at primary care practices associated with MGH, with screening rates for Latinos being lowest at its Chelsea clinic (35 percent) (Percac-Lima et al., 2014). In response, the Chelsea clinic implemented a patient navigation program for colorectal cancer screening in 2007. The clinic hired a full-time Latina navigator who did outreach to the Latino population. She tried to counter many of the barriers to colorectal cancer screening, including transportation, low literacy, lack of fluency in English, inability to take time off work, fear, and a lack of understanding of the importance of screening, according to Oo. "Colorectal cancer screening is not someone's top priority if they have housing and hunger issues, and violence in their community," she said. In addition, several other community health workers, including those from

Somalia, Bosnia, and Arabic-speaking nations, received additional training to help patients with colorectal cancer screening. By 2012, colorectal cancer screening rates were the same at Chelsea as they were for other MGH facilities (Percac-Lima et al., 2014).

Apoyo con Cariño Palliative Care Program

Fischer reported on the Apoyo con Cariño patient navigation study, which is aimed at improving palliative care for Latinos in several counties in Colorado. This research study enrolled 223 Latino adults who had advanced cancer (Fischer et al., 2017). Half of these patients were Spanish speaking and were at or below the poverty line, and nearly half had less than a high school education.

All patients received culturally tailored materials in English or Spanish that focused on different palliative care domains. All of the materials were grounded in core Latino values, such as the importance of taking care of and spending time with family members, which Fischer and her colleagues had previously identified with qualitative surveys of the community. The materials were written at the fifth grade reading level and included pictures so patients with low literacy skills could understand and use them. In addition, a community advisory panel helped the investigators develop and subsequently test the program.

Patients received five home visits from patient navigators, who focused on advanced care planning, pain and symptom management, and hospice care. In addition, navigators helped patients access community resources, and provided emotional and logistical support for families. To "meet patients where they are," navigators engaged with patients and their families on the weekends and at night in their homes, Fischer said. "The navigators understood that people were trying to hold down a job and did not have enough money for rent or food, so they helped decrease that burden instead of adding to it," Fischer said.

Although 55 percent of a control group had spoken to their families about their future health care preferences, 84 percent of those who received the intervention had done so (Fischer et al., 2017). In addition, only 35 percent in the control group had spoken to a clinician about their future health care decisions, versus 60 percent of those in the pilot program. Nearly 70 percent of pilot program participants completed advance directives, according to their charts, whereas only 33 percent of patients in the control group did so. Patients receiving navigation services also reported greater symptom relief than patients in the control group. But there were no significant differences between patients in the intervention and control groups regarding degree of pain severity or interference, or use of hospice care.

Patient Care Connect Program

Meneses reported on PCCP, also known as the Deep South Cancer Navigation Network, and part of The University of Alabama at Birmingham Health System Cancer Community Network. PCCP was funded by a Health Care Innovation Challenge Grant Award from CMS in 2012. The program integrates lay navigation into the health care system, and focuses on older adults with cancer during treatment, survivorship, or end-of-life care. PCCP also focuses on achieving health rather than emphasizing disease, and promotes personal empowerment for patients and caregivers, as well as proactive participation. Priority is given to patients requiring high-acuity care, so most patients participating in PCCP have lung, ovarian, brain, hematologic, or head and neck cancers, or cancers that are metastatic. The program also includes patients with serious concurrent diseases, such as diabetes, heart failure, or chronic obstructive pulmonary disease. All patients are covered by Medicare.

PCCP encompasses 12 cancer centers in five southern states (Alabama, Florida, Georgia, Mississippi, and Tennessee), with a mixture of academic health science centers and hospital-based, affiliated, or private practices. The program has 12 nurse site managers and 40 lay navigators who have at least a bachelor's or master's degree (Rocque et al., 2016). Hired independently by each of the network sites, the navigators are supported by their nurse supervisor, a physician medical director, and an administrative team. The nurse site manager assigns patients to navigators.

To identify patients' needs, the navigators use a distress thermometer, but also have additional questions relevant to the geriatric patients with advanced cancer in the program (Rocque et al., 2016). These questions encompass concurrent illness, informational needs, cognitive changes, spiritual and religious concerns, and quality of life. Distress domains included in the survey are physical, practical, emotional, cognitive, and informational. The most common concerns that patients report are practical, such as transportation or insurance matters, or informational needs, such as wanting information about fatigue and pain. Navigators help patients gather that information by providing informational pamphlets developed by the ACS for lay audiences with low literacy, and by helping patients determine the questions to ask their clinicians.

The PCCP navigators determine patients' needs and address them if they are not severe, and refer patients with high scores on the distress thermometer to a clinician (Rocque et al., 2016) (see Figure 5). Navigators continue to track and coordinate the care of patients referred to clinicians.

Between January 2014 and June 2015, each navigator helped an average of 152 patients per quarter, about half of which were actively navigated. Each navigator enrolled an average of 31 new patients per quarter, involving about three face-to-face or phone contacts on average (Rocque et al., 2016). The navigators are not limited by traditional clinic-based care and can call or visit patients. "There are many different times and ways in which they can see their patients," Meneses said. Annual salaries for the lay navigators range from $33,400 to $42,300 (Rocque et al., 2017).

An analysis of Medicare claims for more than 6,000 non-navigated control patients and more than 6,000 navigated patients between 2012 and 2015 found that the navigated group of patients had significantly lower Medicare costs and health care utilization, including fewer emergency room

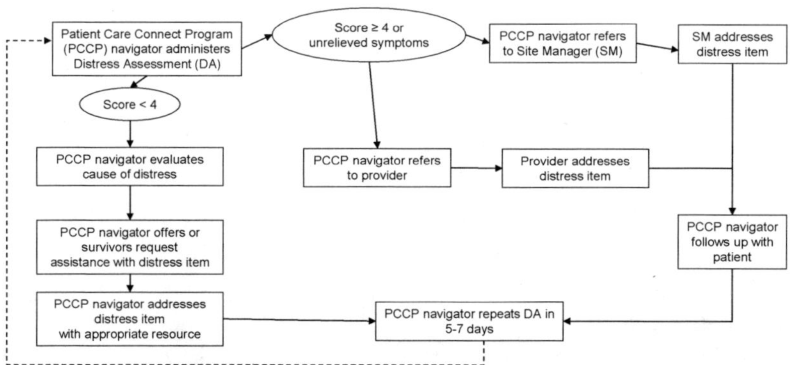

FIGURE 5 Patient Care Connect Program (PCCP) care map.
SOURCES: Meneses presentation, November 13, 2017; Rocque, G. B., E. E. Partridge, M. Pisu, M. Y. Martin, W. Demark-Wahnefried, A. Acemgil, K. Kenzik, E. A. Kvale, K. Meneses, X. Li, Y. Li, K. I. Halilova, B. E. Jackson, C. Chambless, N. Lisovicz, M. Fouad, and R. A. Taylor. *Journal of Oncology Practice* 12(6), 2016:e633–e642. Reprinted with permission.

visits and intensive care unit admissions (Rocque et al., 2017). The total estimated decrease in cost linked to the navigation program was approximately $19 million per year across the whole network (Rocque et al., 2017).

An analysis of these findings estimated a 1 to 10 return on investment, with a reduction in costs of about $475,000 annually for each navigator managing 152 patients per year (Rocque et al., 2017). Meneses said surveys revealed that more than 90 percent of patients' requests for assistance were resolved to the patients' satisfaction. The number of these patient requests declined over time because "the patients increased their own self-management and ability to navigate the system," Meneses said. "This makes a financial case for the sustainability of navigation programs," she stressed, but also added that "without a transition to a values-based payment system, health care systems cannot necessarily implement or expand or even sustain their navigation programs."

Sutter Health Pilot Navigation Program

Cantril reported on the Sutter Health pilot navigation program for breast cancer patients. Sutter Health serves about 27 percent of the California population in 22 northern counties, and has about 13,000 new cancer cases per year, she said. The program is philanthropically endowed and engages nurse navigators and peer support volunteers through the diagnostic, treatment, and posttreatment phases of cancer. The volunteers, who undergo an 8-hour training and monthly staff meetings, mostly offer psychosocial support to patients and families throughout the care trajectory.

Prior to implementing Sutter Health's navigation program, Cantril surveyed clinicians and breast cancer patients on what they wanted from a navigation program. She noted one patient response to the survey was "Do not tell me my diagnosis and then tell me I will get more information from someone with whom I have a future appointment. Give me next steps." The information gathered led her and colleagues to make a nurse navigator available to patients at the time of a suspicious finding to help set up a biopsy. Three days later the patient receives a diagnosis during an in-person appointment with a nurse navigator, at which time next steps are outlined.

Using data in the Sutter Health system, Cantril and her colleagues showed that after the new navigation program was implemented, timeliness of care improved, along with reduced out-migration and increased revenue. Cantril gathered data on one group of patients in the Sutter Health system who did not meet with a nurse navigator until after receiving a cancer diagnosis from a primary care clinician, who then referred them to an oncologist. These data were compared with those of patients who met with a nurse navigator at the time of an abnormal finding. These patients received their breast cancer diagnosis from a nurse navigator, who facilitated their appointment with an oncologist. This comparison revealed that the out-migration to another facility in the first group was 74 percent, while the out-migration of the second group that had been navigated early in the care continuum was 13 to 16 percent. Additional analysis of Sutter Health data suggested that each time a patient with breast cancer leaves the Sutter Health system, there is a loss of about $125,000 in revenue. Given that the annual salary for a nurse navigator there is $125,000, with an additional $44,000 in benefits, retaining only two patients in the health care system through navigation would cover the cost of the navigator, Cantril said.

Blue Distinction® Centers for Cancer Care

Wendy Marinkovich, managing director of the Blue Distinction® Specialty Care Programs at Blue Cross Blue Shield Association, reported on the Blue Distinction® Centers for Cancer Care. This program emphasizes patient-centered coordination of care using an integrated, multidisciplinary delivery model, evidence-based practices, and a commitment to improving the quality and affordability of cancer care (Blue Cross Blue Shield Association, 2017). Health care providers designated under this program are paid under a value-based reimbursement agreement with a local Blue Cross Blue Shield Plan, rather than traditional fee-for-service, with incentives and rewards based on their performance against both quality and cost outcome targets.

This program provides a national framework with consistent selection criteria, and includes all cancer types and care settings. Health care providers that qualify for this designation must meet the program's selection criteria, which may include components that could be facilitated by patient navigation, such as:

- Providing patient caregivers with education about treatment and social work support, resolving language barriers, and communicating the needs and preferences of patients to their clinicians.
- Facilitating timely access to quality medical and psychosocial care from prediagnosis through all phases of the cancer experience.

- Delivering efficient, appropriate, and effective flow of necessary patient care information to clinicians and patients.
- Managing patients throughout all stages of treatment, including survivorship and end-of-life care, and facilitating multidisciplinary care.
- Implementing patient-centered care by including patients and families in planning and goal setting, and by managing symptoms, with the goal of improving the quality of life for both the patient and the family.

In addition, health care providers who qualify for the program's designation must use a standardized Patient Satisfaction and Experience Survey and other measurements to evaluate and improve care delivery.

Geisinger Oncology Navigator Program

Valania described the oncology navigation program of Geisinger, a large nonprofit health care system in rural Pennsylvania. Encompassing 9 hospitals that cover 45 of the 67 counties in Pennsylvania, as well as a few counties in New Jersey, Geisinger has 50 primary care offices, a large system of medical oncology and radiation oncology centers, and about 30,000 employees. Approximately 5,000 new cases of cancer are diagnosed each year throughout the Geisinger system. The for-profit Geisinger Health Plan has a longstanding history of providing a program called the Proven-Health Navigator Services, which includes 120 nurse case managers who are embedded in community practice sites, as well as 26 community health assistants.

Geisinger's oncology-specific navigation program began in late 2010 when it received an NCI Community Cancer Center Program award that enabled it to hire four nurse navigators whose primary purpose was to bridge the gaps in care for patients with cancer in rural areas. These oncology nurse navigators worked in Geisinger primary care sites and connected patients with suspicious findings to appropriate clinicians. But the navigators needed to develop relationships with the clinicians at their sites in order to get patient referrals, she said.

Valania, a social worker, joined the program in 2012 to provide other complex services for patients, including medical assistance, disability applications, psychosocial support, community referrals, mental health assessment, and medical crisis counseling. In addition, nurse navigators were moved from primary care sites to oncology practice settings where there was no navigation support. In 2013, all new oncology patients identified through electronic health records (EHRs) were referred directly to a nurse navigator or a social worker.

There are now five social workers and three nurses providing oncology navigation services within 8 of the 11 medical and radiation oncology sites in Geisinger. Additional nurse, social worker, and lay navigators who do not specialize in oncology also help oncology patients navigate Geisinger's system, and are usually funded and supervised within their own departments. Nurse navigators primarily address medical issues, while social workers focus on financial, transportation, and other practical issues. They also provide emotional support. But as Valania pointed out, "There is an invisible line where one role ends and another begins."

Data collected by Geisinger revealed that patient navigation referrals spiked once navigators were taken out of the primary care setting and placed in oncology practices. In addition, there was a doubling of the number of patient contacts, including phone calls, orders, and letters, as documented in EHRs.

LESSONS LEARNED

Several workshop participants provided examples of lessons learned when designing and implementing a navigation system, including the importance of the following factors:

- Assessing the needs and resources of the community it will serve, making it convenient for patients, and tailoring the program to fit the culture of the communities and individuals served;
- Staffing appropriately and defining the navigator role;
- Building in appropriate metrics and evaluation; and
- Communicating with team members, having program champions, and coordinating and supervising navigators.

Assessing Needs and Resources

Pratt-Chapman suggested defining the patient populations and needs that would be addressed by navigation programs to ensure that services match patient needs, and identifying gaps or bottlenecks in the health care services provided. One should also consider how the program will impact clinicians, and what problems the program would ultimately solve, she added.

"There is not a one-size-fits-all approach to navigation," Burbage stressed. She suggested asking patients, clinicians, and other stakeholders what would help them when developing a new navigation program. "Focus on what is best for the patients in your community and expect growing pains," Burbage added, noting that it may be best to start out small at first, with navigation of patients with certain cancers or during specific parts of the cancer care continuum.

Lathan noted that when the Dana-Farber Cancer Institute developed its patient navigation program, it met with primary care clinicians who provided their input on what the program should entail. "We did not just come in and implement the program. We met with them and asked them 'What do you need, how does it need to be done?'" Lathan said. "That was educational for me because I came in with some ideas of what we should do and found that maybe this is not what they wanted. So we augmented what we wanted to be more like what they wanted. What we found was that not only did the patients love it, but the physicians really liked it as well," Lathan added. He also stressed "knowing your own population that you're interested in, and then making sure that the navigators that are working there know that patient population." Freeman added, "The first question to be asked is 'What does the patient need?' We have to struggle to fit the categories of health care in which we are providers to the needs of the patient and patient navigation."

Melissa Simon said it was important to "understand what actually happens on the ground in clinics." When devising her navigation programs, she and her colleagues conducted citywide assessments of imaging sites, Federally Qualified Health Centers, and community clinics, and undertook an "environmental scan," which involved "following a patient from the time she hits the door of the clinic or imaging center until she leaves, documenting every single process of care," Melissa Simon said.

She also suggested considering the complexities of health care systems at all levels from everyone's viewpoint, including the impact of policies, because "health inequities do not just happen" but are the result of program design, Simon said. Modifying policies "takes a whole lot of education and awareness," she added.

Valania and Blackley suggested conducting a community health needs assessment to determine which problems in the patient community will be navigated. Such an assessment is also one of the requirements for a cancer center to be certified by the CoC, which states, "A patient navigation process, driven by a triennial Community Needs Assessment, is established to address health care disparities and barriers to care for patients. . . . Each calendar year, the patient navigation process is modified or enhanced to address the barrier or additional barriers identified by the Community Needs Assessment," Blackley reported (American College of Surgeons, 2016) (see also the section on Commission on Cancer Standards). She added that such an assessment provides a map or high-level look across the system that can clarify gaps that need to be closed with navigation. Community Needs Assessments also enable input from stakeholders, "so you focus on the biggest area of need, which is critical given limited resources," Blackley said. These assessments also help to provide leverage with a health care system's administration by putting pressure on it to meet the documented needs of its community, Blackley added. The Community Needs Assessment she and her colleagues conducted, for example, revealed the need for financial counselors.

When designing a navigation program, Pratt-Chapman suggested also assessing internal and external resources. Internal resources include funding, space, professional development and training, supervision, and technological infrastructure to support the navigator. External resources include sufficient community-based organizations, and oncology and other specialists to whom the navigator can refer patients. Valania also suggested learning about resources available in the community that will be served by a navigation program so that patients can be referred to those resources. Meneses agreed, noting, "There are strengths in the community that we hadn't necessarily seen or recognized while working at a large acute health care center." Burbage suggested also tapping available informational sources for navigation, such as those published by the Oncology Nursing Society (ONS) or provided by the CoC.

Making Services Convenient for Patients

Narayan stressed that navigation services must be convenient for patients or they will not take advantage of them, as LIVESTRONG discovered when it piloted an in-person service center that cancer patients could come to for support. During the 5-year pilot, LIVESTRONG found that while support services were needed in the community, limited public transportation made them difficult to access. "Convenience is an essential customer service driver and it is even more valuable in health care," Narayan said. LIVESTRONG is now exploring the role technology can play in cancer patient navigation, and is investing time and resources in leveraging technology to increase access to care in a timely manner. For example, it is seeking to increase patient engagement through Web-based interactive tools that are designed to increase patients' sense of empowerment.

Tailoring Services to Fit Community and Individual Needs

Melissa Simon suggested tailoring programs to fit the cultures of the communities that will use them. For example, when developing a navigation program for Chinese immigrants at Mercy Hospital and Medical Center in Chicago, she worked with the local Chinatown community. "We had multiple community talks and conducted all kinds of canvassing to tailor the navigation program correctly for this community to get good outcomes," she said.

Oo said that MGH held focus groups with women from different refugee communities and conducted interviews to assess what would work best with these populations. This outreach suggested that Somali women tended to be comfortable meeting in groups and having group health education sessions, whereas Bosnian women preferred a more individualized approach.

Oo added that on an individual level, it is important to "meet patients where they are. If their issue is hunger, get them referred to a food pantry first and build a trusting relationship with them." Kerber also stressed focusing on what patients need the most. "Find out what are the barriers we need to help work against and go from there," she said.

Fischer suggested tailoring a cancer navigation program to incorporate community views on pain management, palliative care, and end-of-life care. She said focus groups conducted with the Latino community in Colorado revealed that many Latinos there have a fatalistic attitude toward cancer that can hinder them from talking about it or being proactive about their care. Others expressed concern about not wanting to bother their clinicians about their pain. Many members in this community also were initially opposed to the idea of hospice care because they felt dying loved ones should be cared for in the home by their families, and they had the misconception that hospice care involved sending loved ones off to another place to die. But some patients indicated that they preferred to die in the hospital because they did not want to burden their families. Oo stressed that "Even though we can make some generalizations and try to make culturally appropriate materials and interventions, each person has got to be their own voice in their own care plan." Blackley agreed, noting, "You need to have goal-concordant care."

Staffing Appropriately

Oo suggested staffing and matching navigators to patients who speak the same language and have the same ethnic background and religion. "We found it works better that way," Oo said.

Pratt-Chapman suggested staffing health care systems with the types of professionals best suited to meet the navigation needs of the community it serves. "If most of your patients are not adhering to therapies because they're dealing with so much social stress that they are depressed, you should probably be hiring social workers. But if you don't have good symptom management, then you really should start with nurses," Pratt-Chapman said.

Cantril added that it is important to optimize the skills and talents of the health care team appropriately. "I see nurses doing work that someone else could do, physicians doing work that oftentimes nurses can do," Cantril said, giving the example of radiologists charged with conveying breast cancer diagnoses by calling patients when that might be better handled by a patient navigator who meets with the patient.

Who should navigate should also be determined by the level of skills required in a given phase of navigation, and where that phase occurs, Freeman suggested, adding that delivery of navigation services should be cost-effective. "If you're navigating in the community, you bring in community people to help you. Lay navigators can still be in the clinical system, but you also bring in people with professional training, such as nurses and social workers, keeping an eye on the prize—the movement of the patient through the system," Freeman said.

Buescher suggested developing standards for staffing navigation programs to maximize return on investment and other outcomes, and developing and disseminating standard tasks and expectations in navigation, so that all staff can function as navigators in meaningful ways, without relying on a single individual.

Lawrence Shulman, professor and deputy director of clinical services at the University of Pennsylvania Abramson Cancer Center, asked how administrators determine the number of navigators to hire. Buescher responded that there are various approaches, but one way is to document the financial impact on preventing hospital readmissions or reducing no-shows and other outcomes expected from navigation, to determine how many navigators a health care system can afford. He added that there are accountable care organization[13] contracts that reimburse care providers for achieving cancer screening goals, which provide a financial rationale for hiring navigators. In addition, hospitals can conduct a study using their own data to compare the rates of service utilization for navigated patients versus non-navigated patients, essentially calculating the income that navigators could generate for the health care system, and hiring accordingly. "The patient is less likely to leave for a second or third opinion if there is a navigator," he said, giving the example of a University of Minnesota study[14] showing that patients who came back after a second or third opinion cited the navigator as the number one reason for returning.

Defining the Navigator Role

Freeman said navigation should be defined with a clear scope of practice that distinguishes the roles and responsibilities of the navigator from that of other care providers. Blackley noted that a lack of standardization for the navigator role creates confusion that hampers the delivery of quality care for patients. She said when she asks clinicians who are new to her health care system if they have worked with patient navigators before, they often respond, "Yes, but I don't know if my navigator at the other system does what your navigators do." Patients, too, are often confused about the role of the navigator, Blackley added. Pratt-Chapman also suggested clarifying what is expected from navigators, delineating what they should not do, and how they should work with their team members. She warned against hiring navigators to fix the wrong problems. "Navigators cannot fix an inefficient or under-resourced system," Pratt-Chapman said. Burbage suggested defining not only the role of the navigator, but also the role of all team members.

[13] Accountable care organizations "are groups of doctors, hospitals, and other health care providers, who come together voluntarily to give coordinated high quality care to their Medicare patients." See https://www.cms.gov/Medicare/Medicare-Fee-for-Service-Payment/ACO (accessed March 1, 2018).

[14] Unpublished internal analysis conducted in 2006–2007 that followed lung cancer patients at one hospital.

Building in Program Metrics and Evaluation

Several speakers stressed the importance of establishing and deploying a system for tracking the right metrics at the onset of a navigation program to evaluate and document the benefits and cost savings. Buescher suggested documenting return on investment at the local level. Blackley stressed, "We need more information available for those evidence-based practices so we are more able to show the value of navigation and what our navigators are able to do for our patients." She added, "When we all are focused on the same metrics, like those AONN+ [Academy of Oncology Nurse & Patient Navigators] put out, you have strength in numbers." Blackley noted that there are a number of digital tools for tracking metrics. Pratt-Chapman added that programs should specify how evaluation findings will be used to improve the program, and make cancer care simpler and less burdensome for patients.

Melissa Simon suggested creating a bridge between research and practice, using what is learned from on-the-ground community patient navigation implementation experiences to inform future implementation of programs. For example, Melissa Simon noted that she tracks how many women attend community outreach events at health and resource fairs, food pantries, schools, or houses of worship. "We keep counts of how many women we touch within a certain community outreach activity because although a food pantry event may work for one community, it might not be a good strategy for another community," Simon said. Of those women who attend such events, she also tracks how many complete mammogram screening and how many are retained over time by signing them up for mammogram reminder cards.

Wendy Woodward, associate professor and service chief at The University of Texas MD Anderson Cancer Center, asked which metrics are the most important to include in a patient navigation system. Buescher suggested process measures, that is, whether distress screening or pain assessments were done at every visit, and if something adverse was detected, whether it was resolved in a timely way. Pratt-Chapman added that items relevant to cost analyses, such as the number of unplanned hospital admissions, are important, as well as metrics to assess timeliness of care, whether patients are adhering to treatment, and patient-reported outcomes, including satisfaction with care.

Communicating with Team Members

Burbage stressed the importance of communication among navigators, patient advisory councils, and clinicians about what is working with the navigation program and what needs to be improved. McCracken noted that when expanding their patient navigation program, WWC talked with the contractors who were successfully implementing their patient navigation services and then shared those success stories and best practices with other contractors.

Pratt-Chapman also said it was important to increase information sharing across the health care team and to clarify how navigators should communicate with internal and external colleagues, as well as with payers regarding coverage and reimbursement challenges.

Cantril stressed the need for navigators and clinicians to have a respectful dialogue about how to meet patient needs, especially regarding how patients want to receive their cancer diagnosis. Amy Fitzpatrick, general internal medicine physician at the Boston Medical Center, said she thought her patients would rather hear about a cancer diagnosis from her rather than from a navigator they have never met. She said that after she conveys a diagnosis of breast cancer to a patient, a navigator immediately comes into her office and meets with the patient. Fitzpatrick said that this team approach to providing a diagnosis works well.

Cantril also agreed that someone who has had a long-term relationship with a clinician would probably rather receive the diagnosis from that person than from a navigator she or he has just met. But she pointed out that many primary care clinicians at her facility cannot allot the hour of their time that it often takes to properly deliver a cancer diagnosis. Cantril stressed that these primary care clinicians depend on navigators because navigators communicate with radiologists and other clinicians and can expedite patient care. However, she still gives primary care clinicians the option to deliver the cancer diagnosis themselves to patients, and she added that ideally, the primary care clinician and the patient navigator would both be present when conveying a cancer diagnosis and the next steps to be taken.

Valania suggested that patient navigators should "take the time to know your team. Spend 6 months meeting all of the clinicians and making sure you know what their preferences are and how you want to get referrals from them and how they would like for you to do referrals. If you don't have an interpersonal relationship with your team, how are you going to get a warm handoff?" She also added, "You have to have buy-in from the people you work with. If your team does not believe in the navigation work you are doing, it will be very hard to get anything done." Because of the relationships she developed with primary care and oncology clinicians, "I can call someone up and say 'Mr. Smith needs an appointment now' and they give it to me because I've got that relationship," Valania said.

Program Champions

Valania also noted the importance of program champions within her health care system. These champions sustain the program even when resources are scarce. Lathan agreed and said, "This work tends to be personality driven. If the people who are really interested in this leave, who takes it up?" He added that if programs are not institutionalized and in the operational budget, or if a philanthropic donor for the program stops sponsoring it, these programs tend to be dropped. Oo noted that when vacancies recently occurred on her cancer navigation team at MGH, the clinicians in the adult medicine practice at the hospital advocated for filling those vacancies because they realized their productivity, and consequently their salaries, are tied to those navigation services. "It has become such a symbiotic relationship that some of our other departments are chipping in money to support us," Oo said, noting that her navigation services now include an obstetric navigator who helps underserved patients follow through with pre- and postnatal care, which is paid for by the obstetrics and gynecology department at the hospital, rather than by her program or any outside funder.

Coordinating and Supervising Services

Navigation systems require coordination, Freeman stressed. In larger systems of patient care, he said this coordination is best carried out by assigning a navigation coordinator who is responsible for overseeing all phases of navigation activity within a given health care system. "You will never have an Olympic championship relay team unless you have a good coach. Somebody has to be looking at the whole race from beginning to end. The navigators are engaging in phases of the race and are connected together, but the coach is overseeing the whole race," Freeman stressed. Valania also emphasized that supervision of navigators is critical. Pratt-Chapman suggested having clear operational processes and support. Program designs should indicate the protocols, policies, and procedures to follow, as well as who will supervise the navigator and ensure these processes are being followed, she said. She also suggested creating care maps for common problems and seeing if those care maps can be streamlined.

Oo noted that at her facility, a team that includes social workers manages patient navigators and community health workers. These managers provide three types of supervision: (1) administrative supervision, in which navigators are evaluated for whether they are contacting patients, and the results of those contacts; (2) clinical supervision, a manager looks at a patient chart together with a navigator to determine patient barriers and how to break them down; and (3) reflective supervision, which involves meeting weekly with a community health worker or patient navigator to reflect on what they have done with patients, how they feel about it, and whether they took the right approach in a safe and open environment. Oo said that one of the most important forms of supervision provided is reflective supervision.

Choosing a Care Setting

Paul Scribner, senior director of Patient Advocacy Programs at the Aplastic Anemia Center of the Myelodysplastic Syndromes International Foundation, noted that community oncologists sometimes hesitate to refer patients to specialists at a major cancer treatment center due to concerns that these patients will not return for care in the community. "We always suggest that patients go see a specialist who can then work with their community hematologist, but that doesn't always happen," Scribner said.

Lathan agreed, noting that sometimes, "Patients go see the expert and then they don't come back. . . . Let's figure out what is best for the patient and how we can use our individual strengths." Restrictive insurance policies can also limit where patients can be seen for special procedures, such as bone marrow transplants, he added. Melissa Simon responded that regardless of where patients receive their care, the primary care medical home "needs to stay connected with wherever that cancer care is happening and there is a big gap now in care provision and how you do that."

Sometimes patient navigation can help return patients to their primary care facility. Kathleen O'Doherty, a nursing care coordinator for oncology outreach at Main Line Health Cancer Care and the Sidney Kimmel Cancer Center at Jefferson, noted that her job is to help patients navigate between two suburban health care systems in Philadelphia, so that patients benefit from what each system offers. "I follow patients and get them back to their starting place so they don't get lost in the system," O'Doherty said.

NAVIGATION RESOURCES

Several workshop speakers also noted resources and tools that they found helpful for designing patient navigation programs, tracking patients and time spent navigating, conducting distress assessments, deploying telehealth digital tools, and identifying standards for patient navigation.

Program Design

Pratt-Chapman reported that the George Washington University Cancer Center has a free online toolkit for cancer control professionals to advance the field of patient navigation.[15] This toolkit can be used to educate and train patient navigators, provide technical assistance, build navigation coalitions at the state level, and identify policy approaches to sustain patient navigation. Pratt-Chapman also described the George Washington University Cancer Center's road map for cancer control professionals and cancer program administrators, which is a guide for designing a patient navigation process (George Washington University Cancer Center, 2017).

Tracking

Several digital systems can track patients and the time spent by navigators. Lathan said he uses REDCap (Research Electronic Data Capture)[16] to track patients at his facility, while Oo and Valania noted that their health care systems use Epic to document the work of the navigators and to track patients. Blackley reported that her facility developed two informatics systems to help document and collect data. One was developed within the EHRs and tracks the time navigators spend with patients, the navigator reason for contact with the patient, the level of patient navigation acuity, and the primary site of the patient's cancer. "This is information I was able to take back to my administration in order to justify hiring additional full-time employees," Blackley said. She and her colleagues also created a care

---

[15] See https://smhs.gwu.edu/cancercontroltap/resources/advancing-field-cancer-patient-navigation-toolkit-comprehensive-cancer-control (accessed February 26, 2018).

[16] See https://projectredcap.org (accessed March 2, 2018).

management tool that automatically indicates all of a patient's upcoming appointments. It will also alert the navigator in real time if there is a hospital or emergency room admission of a patient, and when the patient was discharged. Such tracking tools are critical when navigators have large patient loads, Blackley stressed.

Pratt-Chapman reported on the free Patient Navigation Barriers and Outcomes Tool (PN-BOT) created by the George Washington University Cancer Center.[17] Based in Excel, this tool includes places to track the amount of time spent navigating specific encounters, patient testimonials, barriers, case management, and other data entry fields. This tool is customizable so it can better meet the needs of a specific program, and has how-to videos for users, Pratt-Chapman noted.

Distress Assessment

To assess the type and severity of patients' needs, several participants reported using the National Comprehensive Cancer Network distress thermometer, but many modified it to include issues relevant to the populations they serve. For an example of modification to the distress thermometer, see the section on PCCP.

Telehealth

Some speakers recommended deploying telehealth digital tools, such as online health care system patient portals, which enable patients to email their clinicians and navigators, receive appointment reminders, or have virtual visits with clinicians. Tony Burns said he found his patient portals at Whitman-Walker Health and the George Washington University Cancer Center to be helpful. Burbage concurred that "there is an opportunity for digital health and innovation and technology." She noted that telehealth might be particularly beneficial for patients who do not have the time to attend in-person meetings. Telehealth could be especially helpful for patient navigation, Burbage said, because much of patient navigation occurs outside of the traditional 9 am-to-5 pm time frame, and it eliminates a lot of time spent playing phone tag with patients. "We have to be available for our patients at the time that works for them, so we need to make it work," she said. Patient navigators in her facility's supportive and palliative care

[17] See https://smhs.gwu.edu/gwci/BarriersTool (accessed February 27, 2018).

program recently started using FaceTime and Skype for meetings with the patients' families, rather than conference call-in lines, because some families were spread out across the country and could not attend in-person meetings.

Standards

Pratt-Chapman, Blackley, and Miller noted several standards for patient navigation, which include the following:

- AONN+ has developed 35 national evidence-based navigation metrics collected from more than 300 source documents that all navigation programs, regardless of the model of navigation chosen, can use to measure success and sustainability (Strusowski et al., 2017);
- AONN+ oncology nurse navigator certification requirements;[18]
- ONS list of oncology nurse navigator core competencies (ONS, 2017);
- CoC *Cancer Program Standards: Ensuring Patient-Centered Care* (American College of Surgeons, 2016);
- George Washington University Cancer Center's *Implementing the Commission on Cancer Standard 3.1 Patient Navigation Process: A Road Map for Comprehensive Cancer Control Professionals and Cancer Program Administrators* (George Washington University Cancer Center, 2017); and
- CoC *National Accreditation Program for Breast Centers Standards Manual.*[19]

PATIENT NAVIGATION COMPETENCIES AND STANDARDS

Navigators have a variety of backgrounds, so establishing competencies for patient navigators creates professional standards and a framework for training, Pratt-Chapman noted. Competencies also clarify the functional importance of a patient navigator to accrediting organizations, payers, funders, and policy makers, she added.

---

[18] See https://www.aonnonline.org/certification/nurse-navigator-certification (accessed February 27, 2018).

[19] See https://www.facs.org/quality-programs/napbc/standards (accessed February 27, 2018).

Paskett said there is also a need for standardized training or certification for navigators, regardless of whether they are lay or nurse navigators, because there are common issues that all navigators need to know how to address. That standardized training or certification occurs should be a benchmark for the Oncology Care Model (OCM) or other cancer care models, Paskett said.

Horn said her own personal experience with cancer made her appreciate the important role of the patient navigator, noting that "you cannot have a navigator in name only. They must have competencies that you measure so they can be absolutely effective, because when they are, they save lives."

McCracken said the Colorado Health Navigator Workforce Development Initiative is developing a credentialing process for health navigator training programs[20] and navigators can take courses from these programs that will be based on a standard set of basic skills. Navigators can then take a competency test and be entered into a registry that employers can use to find and hire patient navigators with the skills and competencies defined by the Initiative.

Kerber added that Georgia CORE works with ACS patient navigators who have training that satisfies national standards, as well as training specific to the Georgia institution at which they are employed.

Brenda Nevidjon, chief executive officer at ONS, noted that there are multiple patient navigation standards because each institution or model system adopts and promotes its own set. "Let's get on the same page. . . . We need to work together and break down these boundaries," she said. Elizabeth Rohan, health scientist at the Centers for Disease Control and Prevention, responded that the National Navigation Roundtable (NNRT) subcommittee focused on the training and education of patient navigators has plans to consider all models in devising their standards. Blackley stressed that "Standardization of navigation is difficult, but now that we have tools available for this through ONS, AONN+, and other organizations, it is important that we build on them and not try to recreate the wheel because that causes confusion in the community."

Burbage noted that many cancer centers are accredited by the CoC and rely on the core competencies specified by the CoC for their patient navigation programs. Most clinical and social worker navigators at cancer centers are required to be certified in oncology, or at least to acquire that

---

[20] See https://www.colorado.gov/pacific/cdphe/health-navigator/credentialing-and-registry (accessed March 12, 2018).

certification within a set amount of time, Burbage added. Tracy Battaglia, associate professor of medicine and epidemiology at the Boston University School of Medicine, said that one possible standard or competency component could be that lay navigators are integrated with other care coordinators and navigators within the health care system.

Commission on Cancer Standards

Miller reported on the American College of Surgeons' CoC standards for cancer navigation services. She noted that the CoC is a consortium of professional organizations dedicated to improving survival and quality of life for cancer patients primarily through setting standards. The CoC recognizes more than 1,500 cancer care programs across the United States that voluntarily meet established standards designed to support delivery of comprehensive, high-quality, multidisciplinary, evidence-based, and patient-centered cancer care.

In 2015, the CoC released for implementation a standard requiring all accredited programs to create a patient navigation process, driven by a triennial Community Needs Assessment that addresses health care disparities and barriers to cancer care. Resources to address identified barriers may be provided either onsite or by referral. The CoC provides technical assistance to help programs complete their Community Needs Assessments.

The Community Needs Assessment drives programs to look inside their community and consider data on cancer incidence and mortality, surveillance, and population statistics, such as gender, age, disability, and other factors that can identify vulnerable populations, Miller noted. It also includes an assessment of cancer-related health factors, such as obesity and smoking rates, as well as social challenges related to transportation, lodging, poverty, educational attainment, and insurance status.

Patient, clinician, and health care system barriers to accessing health care resources and resource gaps identified by the assessment should then be addressed with a plan put forth by the cancer program. Patient barriers might include cost of insurance coverage, language or literacy issues, transportation, child care, housing, or family care, as well as concurrent illnesses or disability, and fears and perceptions that may keep people from seeking care, Miller said. Clinician barriers include time constraints, communication, workforce shortages, reimbursement, and mandated quality care metrics. Health care system barriers include a fragmented system with a lack of shared EHRs, hours of operation that do not cater to the needs of the community, or a difficult-to-reach location of the hospital or clinic.

The strategies that cancer programs develop to meet the needs of the communities they serve should engage community partners and coalitions, Miller stressed. Input from the community can come from patient and clinician surveys and interviews, and from focus groups and public forums, such as town hall meetings. The plans that cancer programs develop should include staff to navigate patients who might otherwise not be able to find and access services. The staff can be patient navigators, social workers, nurses, or other clinicians. "The CoC does not require a patient navigator, but rather, a patient navigation process," Miller said.

The CoC also requires the availability of several patient resources, many of which would fall under the domain or coordination of a patient navigator, including psychosocial services to address patients' psychological, social, spiritual, and financial needs, and pain management programs. The CoC requires patient distress screening, which includes screening patients for anxiety or depression. If those screens are positive, cancer centers must have the ability to refer patients for a more comprehensive psychosocial assessment and the development of an intervention plan. The CoC also requires patients to have a survivorship care plan.

Miller reported that the CoC is currently participating in efforts to create licensing or certification requirements for staff who provide patient navigation services. Future plans include defining and tracking quality metrics and outcomes. As Miller noted, "We are ripe to move to the next phase and look at the cost–benefit information, the staffing structure information, and the competencies that need to be employed to move the marble with patient outcomes. Perhaps in a few years we can strengthen our standard language in some of those ways." Miller said that by formalizing the navigation process and setting standards for cancer programs, "We expect to see positive impacts on patient-related outcomes and progress toward the elimination of cancer disparities in systems across the country."

National Oncology Patient Navigation Competencies

To develop national oncology patient navigation competencies, Pratt-Chapman engaged AONN+, ONS, the National Association of Social Workers, the Association of Oncology Social Work, the Association of

Community Cancer Centers, and on-the-ground patient navigators and community health workers.

After conducting a literature and online search, Pratt-Chapman and her colleagues distilled the competencies shared across the different navigator types. They then conducted focus groups with patient navigators across the country and received input from 22 navigation experts, as well as input from a survey of more than 500 navigators. The final competency list included competencies in eight domains: patient care, knowledge for practice, practice-based learning and improvement, interpersonal and communication skills, systems-based practice, professionalism, interprofessional collaboration, and personal and professional development (Pratt-Chapman et al., 2015). These domains complied with the framework used by the American Association of Medical Colleges and the Accreditation Council for Graduate Medical Education "so we were speaking the same language," Pratt-Chapman said. As a result, competencies for each health care professional role could be delineated within the same overarching domains relevant to any health care professional.

The competencies required for the "patient care" domain included helping patients access cancer care and health care systems by assessing barriers and engaging patients and families in creating potential solutions, as well as being able to assess and identify credible resources and refer out to those resources. Under the "knowledge for practice" domain is a general understanding of cancer and medical terms, health care payment structure and financing, and where to refer patients for answers to questions about insurance coverage and financial assistance.

The "practice-based learning and improvement" domain includes contributing to patient navigation program development, implementation, and evaluation. The "interpersonal and communication skills" domain includes demonstrating empathy, integrity, honesty, and compassion in difficult conversations. But as Pratt-Chapman noted, "It is much harder to figure out how we get these competencies into practice and make sure people are skilled at them, than it is to identify these competencies."

The "professionalism" domain includes applying knowledge of the different roles of clinically licensed and non-licensed professionals and acting within professional boundaries. "Knowing where your job ends and your colleague's begins is important," Pratt-Chapman noted. So is organizing, prioritizing, and being good stewards of resources, which is a competency under the "systems-based practice" domain, she said. The "interprofessional collaboration" domain includes participating in multidisciplinary teams to provide care to patients that is timely, safe, efficient, equitable, and effective. Demonstrating healthy coping mechanisms to respond to stress and employing self-care strategies are competencies under the "personal and professional development" domain.

PATIENT NAVIGATION TRAINING AND CERTIFICATION

Several workshop speakers discussed patient navigation training and certification. Pratt-Chapman described the 20-hour, self-paced, free online training[21] for lay navigators that she developed based on core competencies. This program provides an overview of patient navigation and core competencies, as well as the basics of health care navigation, communication, professionalism, and enhancing practice. The training provides a foundation of knowledge that lay navigators should have, and more training can be added, according to Pratt-Chapman. More than 1,300 patient navigators have enrolled in the training in the first year of its release. The training has also become a core piece of the curriculum of the University of Houston's bachelor-prepared social work program, Pratt-Chapman reported. Other universities and programs are also adopting the training, she said.

Pratt-Chapman also outlined several other online or in-person patient navigation training and certificate programs for nurses or laypeople, most of which charge a fee (Pratt-Chapman and Burhansstipanov, 2018) (see Table 1). These program certificates are provided upon completion of the curriculum. Certification, by contrast, usually involves a proctored examination by a third party different than the one providing the training. "It is a more objective view of whether a person is able to pass a threshold in terms of their abilities and what they know," Pratt-Chapman noted. Currently such certification is provided by AONN+ either for nurse navigators or for non-clinical professional navigators. The National Consortium of Breast Centers also provides navigator certification based on the type of provider, but only for breast programs (Pratt-Chapman and Burhansstipanov, 2018), said Pratt-Chapman.

Pratt-Chapman and her colleagues at the Institute for Patient-Centered Initiatives and Health Equity at the George Washington University Cancer Center are currently piloting a training program called Together-Equitable-

[21] See https://smhs.gwu.edu/cancergate/best-practice/oncology-patient-navigator-training-fundamentals (accessed March 12, 2018) and http://gwcehp.learnercommunity.com/cancer-institute (accessed March 12, 2018).

Accessible-Meaningful (TEAM),[22] in which 24 health care organizations across the country are participating. This no-cost training involves a 5- to 8-hour online component for assessing their organizations and what they wish to change about their cancer care system. This will be followed by 2.5 days at the George Washington University Cancer Center, at which they will receive hands-on technical assistance on troubleshooting and what action steps are needed to achieve their system goals. The Institute will then track participants over 4 months and measure their progress. The training will include how to improve patient–clinician communication and provide equitable care in a culturally sensitive way. This training program will include a Continuing Medical Education component.

Meneses also described the training for lay navigators within PCCP. She said that navigators hired by participating institutions come to a University of Alabama at Birmingham coordination center for a week-long orientation at which they are taught issues related to cancer and cancer care, treatments, symptoms, and side effects. In addition, they are taught how to communicate and work with patients and families, especially when dealing with cancer-related issues such as advanced directives, and how to communicate with care team members. Training involves roleplaying with nurses and site managers, as well as with other lay navigators. Cantril noted that at her facility, volunteer peer navigators undergo an 8-hour training session and attend monthly meetings. Battaglia said that the Massachusetts Department of Public Health Technical Assistance Program also provides training and education support for implementing patient navigation in health care settings. McCracken said a patient navigation training collaborative in Colorado is focused on lay navigators and includes training for the supervisors of navigators. Kerber added that the Georgia CORE also has a lay navigator training program, as well as a train-the-trainer program. The Georgia CORE and the Georgia Society of Clinical Oncology also provide education and other forms of support to cancer patient navigators on a regular basis, she said.

Battaglia pointed out that the NNRT identified training and education as a high priority to ensure consistent competencies among people working as navigators, community health workers, and care coordinators.

---

[22] See https://cancercenter.gwu.edu/for-health-professionals/team-together-equitable-accessible-meaningful (accessed March 1, 2018).

TABLE 1 Professional Certificate Programs

Program	Website	Target Audience	Cost
Cancer Navigator Program	cancernavigatorprogram.org	Social workers, counselors, chaplains, and other staff supporting patients, including navigators	$550
Cancer Navigator Program	cancernavigatorprogram.org	Registered nurses	$550
George Washington University Cancer Center—Oncology Patient Navigator Training: The Fundamentals	bit.ly/GWCCOnlineAcademy	Any navigator	No cost
George Washington University Cancer Center—Executive Training on Navigation and Survivorship	bit.ly/GWCCOnlineAcademy	Supervisors of navigators, program leaders	No cost
Harold P. Freeman Patient Navigation Institute Patient Navigation Program	www.hpfreemanpni.org	Patient navigators	$995

Course Format	Curriculum
Online—21 lessons	• Cancer biology • Prevention and screening methods • Treatment options • Palliative/end-of-life care • Financial resources • Patient education • Advocacy • Resource utilization and support • Spiritual, psychosocial, and emotional support needs • Home health and hospice care • Medicare, Medicaid, and other payers
Online—24 lessons	• All content from general navigator program plus symptom management
Online—20 lessons, interactive, evidence-based with case studies, comes with free online guide	• Overview of patient navigation and core competencies • Basics of health care • Basics of patient navigation • Enhancing communication • Professionalism • Enhancing practice
Online, interactive, evidence-based with case studies and supplemental written content and activities, comes with free online workbook	Nuts and bolts of navigation and survivorship program development, including • Identifying need • Planning your program: models • Components, tools, goal setting, and more • Funding and sustaining your program • Evaluating your program • Creating a business plan
2 days, in-person—10 modules, including patient interaction and case studies	• Curriculum not publicly available • Focus on increased retention, diagnostic, and treatment resolution rates

continued

TABLE 1 Continued

Program	Website	Target Audience	Cost
Misericordia University	www.misericordia.edu/page.cfm?p=1814	Undergraduate students wishing to become navigators	Based on tuition to complete required credits
Native Patient Navigator's Training	www.NatAmCancer.org	Any navigator working with indigenous peoples	$1,100
Otero Junior College	www.ojc.edu/academics/academicprograms/ctehealthnav.aspx	Patient navigators	Based on tuition to complete required credits

Course Format	Curriculum
Bachelor of health science, patient navigation specialization, patient navigation certificate	Helps new navigators guide patients, caregivers, and family members through a treatment plan with the goal of improving patient outcomes: • Values of justice and hospitality • Physical, emotional, and social support to patients following a treatment plan • Communication and interviewing to assess barriers to care • Current health care trends and issues that impact the patient navigators' ability to provide care/assistance • Identify and explain health resources, including publicly funded health insurance programs and health delivery systems
5 days, in-person, learning reinforcement sessions post-training	• American Indian and Alaskan Native history and impact on community member perceptions and health care • Cultural competency, goal setting and culture, navigator safety • Navigating the Health Care Systems and the Indian Health Service Purchased Referred Care • Outreach and education strategies • Communication • Health care team collaboration • Resources • Cancer continuum and tumor-specific education • Clinical trials, confidentiality, Health Insurance Portability and Accountability Act of 1996, data collection and protocols for dissemination • Tribal institutional review boards and approval processes
In-person	• Linking patients with services • Providing information and resources • Helping providers interact with patients • Health education and behavior change promotion

continued

TABLE 1 Continued

Program	Website	Target Audience	Cost
Patient Navigator Training Collaborative	patientnavigatortraining.org	Patient navigators (level 1), experienced patient navigators, nurses, social workers (level 2), administrators (level 3)	Varies
Shenandoah University/Inova Health System	www.su.edu/nursing/certificate-programs/care-navigator-certificate	Registered nurses	$3,000
Smith Center Patient Navigation Training in Integrative Cancer Care	smithcenter.org/institute-for-integrativeoncology-navigation	Navigators interested in integrative care	$995

Course Format	Curriculum
In-person (level 1, 2, 3), online (level 2), special topic webinars	• Level 1—fundamentals: basic patient navigation skills, resources, basic health promotion, professional conduct, motivational interviewing • Level 2—for experienced navigators, nurses, or social workers: includes small group work, roleplay, practice sessions, and group discussion. Real-life scenarios and examples are woven throughout each course • Level 3—supervisors of navigators, program planners, and administrators of patient navigator programs: provides a basic understanding of the patient navigator intervention model, reviews challenges facing program managers, and provides strategies for an effective program. Includes identifying evidence-based clinical guidelines, utilizing registries for identifying patients, developing standard work flows, navigator training, navigator supervision needs, and evaluation of services • E-Learning: Preventive health care 101, introduction to the health care system, introduction to chronic disease, clinical trials and patient navigation, HIV-related cancer research studies • Webinars: Poverty and self-sufficiency, 2013 National Culturally and Linguistically Appropriate Services Standards for patient navigators, basic crisis management skills for patient navigators, managing difficult patient encounters
5 days in-person/ blended learning, 56 contact hours, and a preceptorship	• Assist patients in navigating complex health care services across the continuum of care • Build skills in delivering care coordination services within new health care models and patient settings
2 pre-training teleconferences, 5 days in-person	• Morning yoga at patient navigation training • Client assessment • Difficult conversations • Survivorship issues • The art of healing • Spiritual support • Nutrition • Application of complementary modalities • Building trust • Planning your integrative practice

continued

TABLE 1 Continued

Program	Website	Target Audience	Cost
University of Miami Healthcare Navigator Certificate	continue.miami.edu/en/packagedetail.aspx?p=100	Any navigator or patient advocate	$4,995

SOURCES: Pratt-Chapman presentation, November 13, 2017; Pratt-Chapman and Burhansstipanov, 2018.

EXAMPLES OF POLICY CHALLENGES AND OPPORTUNITIES

Several presenters discussed examples of policy initiatives that could help address key challenges in patient navigation, including making navigation services more affordable, making navigation more of a national priority, and creating a national clearinghouse for patient navigation resources.

Increasing Affordability of Patient Navigation

Direct reimbursement for patient navigation services is not currently available, so it is often financially supported by philanthropic or research grants, volunteer efforts, or institutional resources in large cancer centers. This uneven funding can hinder navigation services from reaching diverse populations and create inequities, said Lisa Kennedy Sheldon, chief clinical officer at ONS. Lathan responded that "If navigation services could be billable, then you could see this being something used not just by centers that have a lot of money and can incorporate navigation into their operation costs, and not just by great researchers funded by grants, but by everybody who needs it."

Paskett suggested finding ways to sustain patient navigation using different models and payment structures. Melissa Simon noted the evolving movement from fee-for-service medical care to pay-for-performance medical care that has been incorporated into OCM. In this pilot program, clinicians can bill for a coordination-of-care fee that pays $160 per month per patient on active treatment. Pratt-Chapman noted the variability in patients' needs for navigation services, and asked, "How do we create an

Course Format	Curriculum
Online	• Health advocacy and the role of the health advocate • Understanding the patient illness experience • Health care communications and professionalism • Ethical issues in health care • Health law • Navigating health care financing • Business as a health care advocate

algorithm so payers are not overpaying, but institutions can take the risk of hiring an adequate number of navigators?"

Ronald Kline, medical officer for the patient care model group at CMS, added that with bundled payment systems used in accountable care organizations, navigation services do not have to be billed because the money saved by reducing emergency room visits and unplanned hospital admissions through navigation services returns to the medical facility as revenue. But those savings cannot usually be applied to pay for navigation services in a fee-for-service medical care system, Kline noted. Miller suggested advocating for inclusion of navigation services in a bundled payment system when evidence indicates the service is needed.

Evans asked what more is required by payers for navigation to be reimbursed, given all of the evidence gathered on the value and return on investment of navigation services to date. Marinkovich responded that while provider payment is determined independently by each local Blue Plan, many Blue Cross Blue Shield Plans are considering providing payment for care coordination to practices and provider groups, but they are focusing on patient-centered care that is well coordinated, not necessarily on the role of a patient navigator. Pratt-Chapman also noted,

> If we try to reimburse for navigation as a service, those patients with better insurance products are going to get the service and not those who need navigation the most. We want to ensure we are not increasing disparities with an innovation, given that institutions with more resources may be able to provide more navigation than those with fewer resources.

Lathan noted that the expanded access to health care enabled by the state of Massachusetts "has helped dramatically and allows us to do some things that other states cannot. However, it has also uncovered that even in a state with 90 to 98 percent insurance coverage, there are still major issues with access—we still have capacity issues and the insurance is helpful, but it doesn't take away the disparities completely." Oo added that even prior to expanded insurance coverage, Massachusetts hospitals have returned some of their tax savings to the community via community benefit guidelines, where they could be used to pay for the medical care of uninsured patients.

Melissa Simon said that in 2015, Illinois passed the Breast Cancer Excellence in Survival and Treatment Act,[23] which provided funding for three patient navigation pilot programs in Illinois. This bill was passed partly based on data she and others in the Metropolitan Chicago Breast Cancer Task Force had collected on the benefits of patient navigation programs, according to Simon.

Making Patient Navigation a Nationwide Priority

Several presenters suggested making patient navigation more of a nationwide priority. Greg Simon stressed that "Patient navigation has got to be a priority of our medical system, and more importantly, it has to be a priority for our society. We are going to have a system in this country for navigating self-driving cars before we have a system for patient navigation. They both will save lives, but patient navigation will save a whole lot more." Horn added that the nation is moving too slowly in making patient navigation a priority, pointing out that evidence of its benefits have been known for some time. "Just do it. We know it pays for itself, even if we cannot totally prove it and more importantly, even if it did not fund itself, do our patients deserve any less? If it was your wife, son, or daughter, do you want them to have a navigator?" Horn asked. But Melissa Simon also stressed that "Patient navigators are not Band-Aids. They are part of the solution, but you cannot just put a patient navigator into a broken health system and expect it to work."

Greg Simon noted that one reason patient navigation has not been made more of a priority is because most people are unaware of the gaps in the health care system that navigation addresses until they suffer a health care crisis themselves. "We are trying to create the system that patients

---

[23] Public Act Number 99-0433. See http://www.ilga.gov/legislation/BillStatus.asp?DocTypeID=HB&DocNum=3673&GAID=13&SessionID=88&LegID=89870 (accessed March 1, 2018).

think we already have. Patients assume that their doctors will collaborate with other doctors and other hospitals, and that there is a system to help them pay their expenses, watch their kids, and even pay for their parking, but there is not," he said. Even Vice President Joe Biden had a hard time navigating the health care system when his son was diagnosed with a brain tumor, he said.

One way to make patient navigation more of a nation- or statewide priority is to engage public health departments, several presenters said. McCracken said the Colorado Department of Public Health and Environment focuses their patient navigation efforts on the individuals from communities less likely to be screened and more likely to have poorer outcomes. The department also supports the clinic quality improvement activities of organizations and other activities that support navigation. Such activities can include creating policies, procedures, and workflows for addressing cancer screenings and patient navigation. In addition, at the community level, public health organizations can conduct outreach to populations less likely to be screened for cancers and help them access such screening at clinics, McCracken noted. Rohan said, "If there are clinics trying to reach the hardest to reach, collaborating with public health might be a way to help them."

Kerber added that in Georgia there are nurse-staffed health centers in every county. "People can just walk into their local health center to get their care or have their questions answered with clinicians that many of them have grown up with," she said, noting these community clinics offer an opportunity to connect on the community level, which often makes the screenings and other care they offer more amenable to the people they serve.

Battaglia said the Massachusetts Department of Public Health has an Office of Community Health Workers with the focus of increasing the capacity of both the community and the health systems to do patient navigation in the field. This office offers trainings[24] and "sets the tone" for competency training in the state, according to Battaglia, and also has a technical assistance arm that enables health systems to integrate and implement evidence-based navigation programs.

---

[24] See http://www.mass.gov/eohhs/gov/departments/dph/programs/community-health/prevention-and-wellness/comm-health-wkrs/chw-training-resources.html (accessed March 1, 2018).

National Navigation Resource Clearinghouse

Cantril suggested creating a national navigation clearinghouse of resources that could include a centralized orientation program so every program "wouldn't have to reinvent the wheel" and could build on the resources that others developed. Pratt-Chapman noted that the George Washington University Cancer Center has a website called Generation and Translation of Evidence (GATE),[25] but it has had limited uptake. GATE was designed to facilitate communication among clinicians, researchers, and patients, "but the clinicians and navigators tend to underestimate what they can contribute and are so stretched for time [that] they find it hard to draft and submit something," Pratt-Chapman said. Miller added that the CoC has also experienced limited uptake when it asked all of its accredited programs, more than 1,500, to submit resources, best practices, and ideas. She added that the Comprehensive Cancer Control National Partnership[26] is a nationally based coalition that tries to gather resources on certain topics and has had some success in this regard. Woodward noted that uptake for a national navigation resource clearinghouse might depend on demand because it is easier to share resources online at one website rather than individually. Blackley commented that she was surprised to hear there was not much uptake, and Pratt-Chapman responded, "People don't realize that they have valuable information that other people could benefit from."

RECENT POLICY INITIATIVES IN PATIENT NAVIGATION

A number of workshop speakers reported on several recent patient navigation policy initiatives, including OCM, the Cancer Moonshot and Biden Cancer Initiative, and the NNRT.

Oncology Care Model

Buescher described OCM, a CMS demonstration program involving approximately 190 practices aimed at improving the quality of cancer care outcomes, the patient experience, and the overall cost of care. The 5-year pilot project has an innovative payment model with bundled payments for episodes of care surrounding chemotherapy administration to cancer

[25] See https://smhs.gwu.edu/cancergate (accessed March 1, 2018).

[26] See https://www.cccnationalpartners.org (accessed March 1, 2018).

patients, which financially incentivizes high-quality, coordinated care. Participating practices must adhere to certain care transformation requirements, one of which is providing the core functions of patient navigation, with reimbursement of $160 per month per patient on active treatment. These core functions are defined as follows:

- Coordinating appointments with providers for timely diagnostic and treatment services;
- Maintaining communication with patients, survivors, families, and providers to monitor patient experience;
- Ensuring appropriate medical records are available at appointments;
- Arranging language translation services if needed;
- Facilitating follow-up services and providing access to clinical trials; and
- Building partnerships with local agencies and groups.

OCM participants also must have metrics for quality improvement. Some of these metrics are related to patient navigation and include hospital and emergency room admission rates, screening for depression and pain and developing a plan for addressing them if they occur, and documenting end-of-life preferences. Another quality measure is the Consumer Assessment of Healthcare Providers and Systems Cancer Care Survey, which assesses how the care team interacts with the patient, and how satisfied patients were with their health care experience (AHRQ, 2017). Determining if care is patient-centered is the general aim of this survey, which includes questions related to patient navigation, such as symptom management, access to care, shared decision making, and whether providers listened to patients and provided clear instructions. Such metrics, requirements, and other incentives under OCM aim to promote more clinician engagement with patients, Buescher noted.

Buescher reported on how the Ann B. Barshinger Cancer Institute, a medium-sized community hospital cancer institute in rural Pennsylvania, modified its practices to meet the requirements of OCM. "The challenge with OCM is that we have to prove we are actually navigating patients," Buescher noted. The OCM navigation requirements were mostly met by assigning these responsibilities to existing staff, including patient navigators, schedulers, and a clinical trials nurse. Additional patient navigators and schedulers were hired to coordinate appointments with clinicians, and the OCM standards were made clear to all nine cancer disease teams. These teams have daily huddles to prioritize patient issues and determine who will manage them and how. Navigators play an important role in reporting back to the disease teams about "whether this process is working for patients as a whole, and that helps us identify and prioritize what the issues are," Buescher said. Patients are ranked according to their diagnosis and cancer stage, concurrent illnesses, and behavioral, cultural, financial, educational, and societal factors that might influence their care. This ranking prioritizes which patients to focus on first and determines how much navigation they should receive (see Figure 6).

The cancer program also started using standardized templates for advanced care plans, for shared decision making, and for devising treatment plans. These plans are not only documented in their EHR system, but are also printed out and shared with everyone on the care team, including other referring specialists and primary care clinicians. These templates were written to be easily understood by patients, and clinicians were trained in how to use them. There are also standardized symptom management plans. Additional information technology support helped adapt the EHR system to these new practices.

Because everything is tracked in real time, data on how well clinicians are achieving various objectives can be graphically displayed and presented weekly, so they can focus on areas for improvement. "Instead of doing a

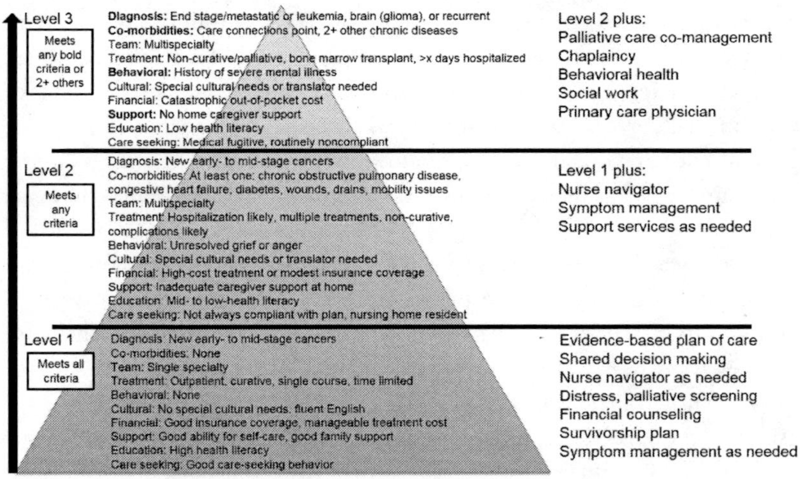

FIGURE 6 Lancaster General Health risk-based care model.
SOURCE: Buescher presentation, November 13, 2017.

retrospective quality review out of our cancer registry on care that took place 9 months ago, we are giving physicians a view of what happened last week and specifying what tasks they need to do at the next appointment to get a perfect quality score next month," Buescher said.

Since the new OCM procedures and processes were instituted in 2016, the cancer institute has seen improvement in a number of quality metrics, including fewer emergency room visits and an increase in the number of patients who had a discussion on or completed advanced care planning with their clinicians. The number screened for depression and pain also increased. Patient satisfaction was in the 90th percentile. Those improvements were accompanied by a large decrease in the amount of money Medicare spent for each beneficiary treated at the facility. Buescher also said that participating in the OCM model improved teamwork and morale, and fostered a culture of rapid process improvement and innovation.

Buescher attributed his cancer institute's OCM success to a number of factors, including high levels of staff and clinician engagement, process improvement training, protected time for clinicians and staff to work on performance improvement projects, and focused leadership attention. Buescher concluded that OCM "helps recalibrate everybody toward shared goals that are good for both the providers and patients."

Robert Green, senior vice president of clinical oncology at Flatiron Health, noted that Flatiron Health, which provides software for oncology clinicians, tailored their software so it conveniently shows in one place all of the quality measures required from participants of OCM. Also included in their software are algorithms and rules within the EHR that identify and track which patients are eligible for OCM bundled payments. "We think we are making progress using technology to help make something that is critically important for patients a little bit easier and more efficient within the practices," Green said.

Cancer Moonshot/Biden Cancer Initiative

Greg Simon said that the goal of the Biden Cancer Initiative, formerly the Cancer Moonshot program, is to "develop and drive implementation of solutions to accelerate progress in cancer prevention, detection, diagnosis, research, and care, and to reduce disparities in cancer outcomes" (Biden Cancer Initiative, 2018). In 2016, Congress authorized funding for the Cancer Moonshot for 7 years (NCI, 2018). By January 2017, the Cancer

Moonshot had launched nearly 80 new actions and collaborations (Preston, 2017).

A major focus of the program is to make cancer care more patient- centered, data rich, and collaborative, Greg Simon noted. "There is no technical problem for any of the issues we are dealing with—data standards and sharing, clinical trial reform, and patient navigation are all within our grasp. It is all about attitude and culture. That is why we all have to band together to change," Simon said. He suggested that the Biden Cancer Initiative could help on a policy level to further cancer patient navigation, "whether it is federal reimbursement or convincing hospitals and cancer centers that your mission is to help patients, not to make money, and that if you help patients, you will make money."

Simon added that as part of the Biden Cancer Initiative, it would be worthwhile to bring together clinicians and experts versed in technology to devise apps and other digital technologies to aid patient navigation. "There are thousands of companies working on apps to do all kinds of things, but the question remains—why do we not know what is going on with the patients we are trying to help?" Simon explained.

National Navigation Roundtable

Battaglia reported on the NNRT, which was launched in 2017 and is sponsored by the ACS. The NNRT is a national coalition of more than 40 members, organizations, and individuals who are dedicated to achieving health equity and access to quality care across the cancer continuum. Its goal is to advance navigation efforts that eliminate barriers to cancer care, reduce disparities in health outcomes, and foster ongoing health equity. As Battaglia noted, "the NNRT brings people together from the public and private sectors, and from the medical and civic communities, to have a unified voice and to leverage their talents to move a process forward."

The NNRT focuses on three major areas:

1. Evidence-based, promising practices that aim to establish an outcome-driven patient navigation model;
2. Training and certification that aim to ensure there is a trained workforce to implement the model; and
3. Developing and supporting policy effects that favor paying for the patient navigation model.

All three task groups agree that "we really need to be making the business case for how we take patient navigation and make it a sustainable model. We need the right metrics, competencies, and trainings, and we need the right policies in place for us to be able to do that," Battaglia said.

WORKSHOP WRAP-UP

Shulman asked why, given all of the evidence of benefits of patient navigation that has been shown since the 1980s, "are we still struggling with trying to develop a robust approach to patient navigation for cancer patients in the United States? You have to ask the right questions and if we don't, we are not going to end up in the right place."

Given that there are always resource constraints, navigation targeted to those patients who need it the most is likely to be the right place to start, Shulman noted, but added, "If you are the vice president of the United States and you need navigation for your son, there is a message there." He suggested starting with targeted navigation, but eventually health care facilities should strive to offer navigation for everyone. "I have not heard of anybody who is not going to benefit from it," he said.

Noting all of the different models for providing patient navigation, Shulman stressed that there probably is not one ideal model. "The programs look a bit different because the needs are different and they should be created around the needs and not necessarily around the notion that everybody should have exactly the same model," he said. However, that should not preclude providing standard definitions, training, and certification for patient navigators, which need to be explored more, he said.

He stressed the difference between a navigator and a navigator program at a health care facility, and suggested that both are needed for a navigator to work effectively. "Navigators may fill some of the cracks in a system, but they cannot be expected to fix systems that are truly broken. We need to make sure our systems are facilitating the work of navigators so they can truly bridge some of those gaps."

With regard to making a business case for patient navigation, Shulman noted that "everything lines up in the same direction—you have increased patient retention that is good for your bottom line; you have decreased resource utilization, which can translate into a better bottom line if you are in a program like OCM. And yet it is very hard to convince hospital systems to write that initial check and hire navigators, even though the return on investment will pay for their salary and benefits.... Something is missing in that equation."

To help make the business case, Shulman suggested collecting more outcomes, such as patient satisfaction, patient engagement with care, complication rates, costs, and survival rates. "I don't think we will get to where we need to go unless we can show these outcomes," he said. Even the CoC, which has made patient navigation a requirement of their accreditation, "struggles with whether navigation programs are effective [components] that are changing outcomes or just a box that is checked," Shulman said. "It is a struggle for our accreditation staff as they go around to 1,500 hospitals to really know in a day's site visit what is going on," he said. But he stressed that the patient navigation requirement is a lever for change, and that payers can also provide a big lever. He noted the "visionary direction" that the Blue Cross Blue Shield Foundation is taking through its Blue Distinction® program to encourage hospital administrators to provide value-based care. "Government and private payers can have a lot of influence in driving care," Shulman said.

Shulman emphasized, "The only way we are going to make progress is if the National Navigation Roundtable, the payers, the Commission on Cancer, and the National Cancer Policy Forum work together to change the culture in this country to do what our patients really need us to do."

REFERENCES

ACS (American Cancer Society). 1989. A summary of the American Cancer Society report to the nation: Cancer in the poor. *CA: A Cancer Journal for Clinicians* 39(5):263–265.

AHRQ (Agency for Healthcare Research and Quality). 2017. *CAHPS cancer care survey.* https://www.ahrq.gov/cahps/surveys-guidance/cancer/index.html (accessed February 27, 2018).

American College of Surgeons. 2016. *Cancer program standards: Ensuring patient-centered care,* https://www.facs.org/~/media/files/quality%20programs/cancer/coc/2016%20coc%20standards%20manual_interactive%20pdf.ashx (accessed February 23, 2018).

Basu, M., J. Linebarger, S. G. A. Gabram, S. G. Patterson, M. Amin, and K. C. Ward. 2013. The effect of nurse navigation on timeliness of breast cancer care at an academic comprehensive cancer center. *Cancer* 119(14):2524–2531.

Biden Cancer Initiative. 2018. *Mission.* https://bidencancer.org/#mission (accessed March 1, 2018).

Blue Cross Blue Shield Association. 2016. *Blue distinction centers for cancer care selection criteria.* https://www.bcbs.com/sites/default/files/file-attachments/page/Cancer.Care_.Selection.Criteria.pdf (accessed March 9, 2018).

Blue Cross Blue Shield Association. 2017. *Blue distinction centers for cancer care.* https://www.bcbs.com/sites/default/files/file-attachments/page/BCBS.BlueDistinctionSpecialtyCare.ProgramOverview.pdf (accessed March 9, 2018).

Boston Public Health Commisstion. 2013. *Health of Boston 2012-2013: A neighborhood focus.* http://www.bphc.org/healthdata/health-of-boston-report/Documents/HOB-2012-2013/HOB12-13_FullReport.pdf (accessed February 27, 2018).

Faris, N., X. Yu, S. Sareen, R. S. Signore, L. M. McHugh, K. Roark, E. T. Robbins, and R. U. Osarogiagbon. 2015. Preoperative evaluation of lung cancer in a community health care setting. *The Annals of Thoracic Surgery* 100(2):394–400.

Fischer, S., S. Min, D. Kline, and R. Fink. 2017. Apoyo con Cariño: Patient navigation to improve palliative care outcomes for Latinos with advanced cancer. *Journal of Pain and Symptom Management* 53(2):396–397.

Freeman, H. P. 1989. Cancer in the socioeconomically disadvantaged. *CA: A Cancer Journal for Clinicians* 39(5):266–288.

Freeman, H. P. 2001. *Voices of a broken system: Real people, real problems, president's cancer panel: Report of the chairman.* https://deainfo.nci.nih.gov/advisory/pcp/archive/pcp00-01rpt/PCPvideo/voices_files/PDFfiles/PCPbook.pdf (accessed February 23, 2018).

Freeman, H. P. 2006. Patient navigation: A community centered approach to reducing cancer mortality. *Journal of Cancer Education* 21(1 Suppl):S11–S14.

Freeman, H. P. 2012. The origin, evolution, and principles of patient navigation. *Cancer Epidemiology, Biomarkers & Prevention* 21(10):1614.

Freeman, H. P., and R. L. Rodriguez. 2011. The history and principles of patient navigation. *Cancer* 117(15):3539–3542.

Freeman, H. P., and T. J. Wasfie. 1989. Cancer of the breast in poor black women. *Cancer* 63(12):2562–2569.

Freeman, H. P., B. J. Muth, and J. F. Kerner. 1995. Expanding acccss to cancer screening and clinical follow-up among the medically underserved. *Cancer Pract* 3(1):19–30.

Freund, K. M., T. A. Battaglia, E. Calhoun, J. S. Darnell, D. J. Dudley, K. Fiscella, M. L. Hare, N. LaVerda, J.-H. Lee, P. Levine, D. M. Murray, S. R. Patierno, P. C. Raich, R. G. Roetzheim, M. Simon, F. R. Snyder, V. Warren-Mears, E. M. Whitley, P. Winters, G. S. Young, E. D. Paskett, and Writing Group of the Patient Navigation Research Program. 2014. Impact of patient navigation on timely cancer care: The patient navigation research program. *Journal of the National Cancer Institute* 106(6):dju115.

George Washington University Cancer Center. 2017. *Implementing the commission on cancer standard 3.1: Patient navigation process.* https://cancercenter.gwu.edu/sites/default/files/coc_navigation_standard_road_map.pdf (accessed March 9, 2018).

Gordils-Perez, J., S. Schneider, M. Gabel, and K. Trotter. 2017. Oncology nurse navigation: Development and implementation of a program at a comprehensive cancer center. *Clinical Journal of Oncology Nursing* 21(5):581–588.

Harding, M. M., and S. McCrone. 2013. Experiences of non-navigated women undergoing breast diagnostic evaluation. *Clinical Journal of Oncology Nursing* 17(1):E8–E12.

Hirschman, J., S. Whitman, and D. Ansell. 2007. The black:white disparity in breast cancer mortality: The example of Chicago. *Cancer Causes and Control* 18(3):323–333.

Hunnibell, L. S., M. G. Rose, D. M. Connery, C. E. Grens, J. M. Hampel, M. Rosa, and D. C. Vogel. 2012. Using nurse navigation to improve timeliness of lung cancer care at a veterans hospital. *Clinical Journal of Oncology Nursing* 16(1):29–36.

Hunt, B. R., S. Whitman, and M. S. Hurlbert. 2014. Increasing black:white disparities in breast cancer mortality in the 50 largest cities in the United States. *Cancer Epidemiology* 38(2):118–123.

Katz, M. L., G. S. Young, P. L. Reiter, T. A. Battaglia, K. J. Wells, M. Sanders, M. Simon, D. J. Dudley, S. R. Patierno, and E. D. Paskett. 2014. Barriers reported among patients with breast and cervical abnormalities in the patient navigation research program: Impact on timely care. *Women's Health Issues* 24(1):e155–e162.

Kowalkowski, M. A., D. Raghavan, K. Blackley, V. Morris, and C. Farhangfar. 2016a. Patient navigation associated with decreased 30-day all-cause readmission. *Cancer Epidemiology, Biomarkers & Prevention* 25(3):558.

Kowalkowski, M., D. Raghavan, K. Blackley, V. Morris, and C. J. Farhangfar. 2016b. 12 month survival for oncology patients with versus without patient navigation. *Journal of Clinical Oncology* 34(15 Suppl.):6510.

Krebs, L. U., L. Burhansstipanov, S. Watanabe-Galloway, N. L. Pingatore, D. G. Petereit, and D. Isham. 2013. Navigation as an intervention to eliminate disparities in American Indian communities. *Seminars in Oncology Nursing* 29(2):118–127.

Krok-Schoen, J. L., B. M. Brewer, G. S. Young, R. C. Weier, C. M. Tatum, C. R. DeGraffinreid, and E. D. Paskett. 2015. Participants' barriers to diagnostic resolution and factors associated with needing patient navigation. *Cancer* 121(16):2757–2764.

Krok-Schoen, J. L., J. M. Oliveri, and E. D. Paskett. 2016. Cancer care delivery and women's health: The role of patient navigation. *Frontiers in Oncology* 6:2.

McLaughlin, J. M., R. T. Anderson, A. K. Ferketich, E. E. Seiber, R. Balkrishnan, and E. D. Paskett. 2012. Effect on survival of longer intervals between confirmed diagnosis and treatment initiation among low-income women with breast cancer. *Journal of Clinical Oncology* 30(36):4493–4500.

Morrison, R. S., S. Wallenstein, D. K. Natale, R. S. Senzel, and L. L. Huang. 2000. "We don't carry that"—failure of pharmacies in predominantly nonwhite neighborhoods to stock opioid analgesics. *New England Journal of Medicine* 342(14):1023–1026.

NCI (National Cancer Institute). 2018. *Cancer Moonshot*. https://www.cancer.gov/research/key-initiatives/moonshot-cancer-initiative (accessed February 23, 2018).

Oluwole, S. F., A. O. Ali, A. Adu, B. P. Blane, B. Barlow, R. Oropeza, and H. P. Freeman. 2003. Impact of a cancer screening program on breast cancer stage at diagnosis in a medically underserved urban community. *Journal of the American College of Surgeons* 196(2):180–188.

ONS (Oncology Nursing Society). 2017. *2017 oncology nurse navigator core competencies*. https://www.ons.org/sites/default/files/2017ONNcompetencies.pdf (accessed February 27, 2018).

Percac-Lima, S., J. M. Ashburner, B. Bond, S. A. Oo, and S. J. Atlas. 2013. Decreasing disparities in breast cancer screening in refugee women using culturally tailored patient navigation. *Journal of General Internal Medicine* 28(11):1463–1468.

Percac-Lima, S., L. López, J. M. Ashburner, A. R. Green, and S. J. Atlas. 2014. The longitudinal impact of patient navigation on equity in colorectal cancer screening in a large primary care network. *Cancer* 120(13):2025–2031.

Pratt-Chapman, M., and L. Burhansstipanov. 2018. Navigation training, tools and resources. In *Team-based oncology care: The pivotal role of oncology navigation*, edited by L. D. Shockney. Cham, Switzerland: Springer International Publishing.

Pratt-Chapman, M., A. Willis, and L. Masselink. 2015. Core competencies for oncology patient navigators. *Journal of Oncology Navigation Survivorship* 6(2):16–21.

Preston, J. 2017. *For the Cancer Moonshot, collaboration is still the number one fuel.* https://medcitynews.com/2017/07/cancer-moonshot-collaboration-is-fuel (accessed March 1, 2018).

Reuland, D. S., A. T. Brenner, R. Hoffman, A. McWilliams, R. L. Rhyne, C. Getrich, H. Tapp, M. A. Weaver, D. Callan, L. Cubillos, B. Urquieta de Hernandez, and M. P. Pignone. 2017. Effect of combined patient decision aid and patient navigation vs. usual care for colorectal cancer screening in a vulnerable patient population: A randomized clinical trial. *JAMA Internal Medicine* 177(7):967–974.

Rocque, G. B., E. E. Partridge, M. Pisu, M. Y. Martin, W. Demark-Wahnefried, A. Acemgil, K. Kenzik, E. A. Kvale, K. Meneses, X. Li, Y. Li, K. I. Halilova, B. E. Jackson, C. Chambless, N. Lisovicz, M. Fouad, and R. A. Taylor. 2016. The patient care connect program: Transforming health care through lay navigation. *Journal of Oncology Practice* 12(6):e633–e642.

Rocque, G. B., M. Pisu, B. E. Jackson, E. A. Kvale, W. Demark-Wahnefried, M. Y. Martin, K. Meneses, Y. Li, R. A. Taylor, A. Acemgil, C. P. Williams, N. Lisovicz, M. Fouad, K. M. Kenzik, E. E. Partridge, and Patient Care Connect Group. 2017. Resource use and Medicare costs during lay navigation for geriatric patients with cancer. *JAMA Oncology* 3(6):817–825.

Rodday, A. M., S. K. Parsons, F. Snyder, M. A. Simon, A. A. Llanos, V. Warren-Mears, D. Dudley, J. H. Lee, S. R. Patierno, T. W. Markossian, M. Sanders, E. M. Whitley, and K. M. Freund. 2015. Impact of patient navigation in eliminating economic disparities in cancer care. *Cancer* 121(22):4025–4034.

Samaras, A. T., K. Murphy, N. J. Nonzee, R. Endress, S. Taylor, N. Hajjar, R. Bularzik, C. Frankovich, X. Dong, and M. A. Simon. 2014. Community–campus partnership in action: Lessons learned from the DuPage County patient navigation collaborative. *Progress in Community Health Partnerships: Research, Education, and Action* 8(1):75–81.

Strusowski, T., E. Sein, and D. Johnston. 2017. Academy of oncology nurse & patient navigators announces standardized navigation metrics. *Journal of Oncology Navigation and Survivorship* 8(2):62–68.

Treiman, K., C. Bann, L. Squiers, B. Hemingway, S. R. Arvey, E. Eargle, and R. Rechis. 2015. Cancer support services outside of clinical settings: An evaluation of LIVESTRONG Foundation's cancer navigation program. *Journal of Oncology Navigation and Survivorship* 6(3):8–17.

Urrea, N. M. 2009. *Patient Navigator Outreach and Chronic Disease Prevention Act of 2005*: A bipartisan approach to improving access to care and addressing health disparities. *Health Policy Newsletter* 22(2):1.

Waldman, L. T., L. Svoboda, B. F. Young, G. A. Abel, S. Berlin, A. A. Elfiky, R. A. Freedman, M. Drews, L. Holland, and C. S. Lathan. 2013. A novel community-based delivery model to combat cancer disparities. *Healthcare* 1(3):123–129.

Whitman, S., D. Ansell, J. Orsi, and T. Francois. 2011. The racial disparity in breast cancer mortality. *Journal of Community Health* 36(4):588–596.

Zammitti, E. P., R. A. Cohen, and M. E. Martinez. 2017. *Health insurance coverage: Early release of estimates from the National Health Interview Survey, January–June 2017*. https://www.cdc.gov/nchs/data/nhis/earlyrelease/insur201711.pdf (accessed March 1, 2018).

Appendix A

Statement of Task

An ad hoc committee will plan and host a 1.5-day public workshop that will examine the optimal conditions and components for a successful patient navigation program in oncology. The workshop will feature invited presentations and panel discussions on topics that may include

- stakeholder perspectives on the rationale for and appropriate role of navigation programs;
- how patients access and use navigation programs;
- how target population, setting, and resources influence program design;
- models of navigation programs through the full spectrum of cancer care; and
- potential ways to address knowledge gaps to improve the implementation and effectiveness of navigation programs.

The committee will develop the agenda for the workshop sessions, select and invite speakers and discussants, and moderate the discussions. A proceedings of the presentations and discussions at the workshop will be prepared by a designated rapporteur in accordance with institutional guidelines.

Appendix B

Workshop Agenda

November 13, 2017

7:30 am **Registration**

8:00 am **Welcome from the National Cancer Policy Forum and an Overview of the Workshop**
Lisa Kennedy Sheldon, Oncology Nursing Society
Planning Committee Co-Chair

8:15 am **Session 1: Overview of Patient Navigation**
Moderator: Lawrence Shulman, University of Pennsylvania

Historical Perspective of Patient Navigation and a Vision for the Future

- Harold P. Freeman, Harold P. Freeman Patient Navigation Institute

The Evidence Base for Patient Navigation

- Electra Paskett, The Ohio State University

Navigator Perspective

- Darcy Burbage, Christiana Care Health System

Cancer Survivor Perspectives on Patient Navigation
- Doris Burns, Cancer Survivor
- Tony Burns, Cancer Survivor, Peer Mentor, and Advocate

Panel Discussion

10:15 am Break

10:30 am Session 2: Panel Discussion: Best Practices and Exemplars of Patient Navigation
Moderator: Elizabeth Rohan, Centers for Disease Control and Prevention

- Tracy Battaglia, Boston University School of Medicine
- Amy Bertrand, American Cancer Society
- Alice Kerber, Georgia Center for Oncology Research and Education
- Kris McCracken, Colorado Department of Public Health and Environment
- Aditi Narayan, LIVESTRONG Foundation
- Raymond Osarogiagbon, Baptist Cancer Center

Group Discussion

12:30 pm Lunch

1:15 pm Session 3: Extending the Reach of Patient Navigation Programs to Address Health Disparities: Innovations and Next Steps
Moderator: Lisa Kennedy Sheldon, Oncology Nursing Society

- Stacy Fischer, University of Colorado Denver
- Christopher Lathan, Dana-Farber Cancer Institute/ Harvard Medical School
- Sarah Oo, Massachusetts General Hospital's Chelsea HealthCare Center
- Melissa Simon, Northwestern University Feinberg School of Medicine

Panel Discussion

3:15 pm **Break**

3:30 pm **Session 4: Patient Navigation Program Standards, Metrics, and Quality Improvement Efforts**
Moderator: Wendy Woodward, The University of Texas MD Anderson Cancer Center

Commission on Cancer's Standards and Metrics for Patient Navigation Programs
- Nina Miller, Commission on Cancer

Workforce Competencies in Patient Navigation
- Mandi Pratt-Chapman, George Washington Cancer Center

Centers for Medicare & Medicaid Services Oncology Care Model Standards for Patient Navigation
- Nikolas Buescher, Penn Medicine/Lancaster General Health

Approaches to Quality Improvement in Patient Navigation
- Kris Blackley, Levine Cancer Institute

Panel Discussion

5:30 pm **Wrap-Up Day 1**
Lawrence Shulman, University of Pennsylvania
Planning Committee Co-Chair

November 14, 2017

7:30 am **Registration**

8:00 am **Session 5: Improving Financing and Sustainability of Patient Navigation Programs**
Moderator: Lawrence Shulman, University of Pennsylvania

Financing and Cost-Effectiveness of Patient Navigation Programs

- Karen Meneses, The University of Alabama at Birmingham Comprehensive Cancer Center

Demonstrating Impact and Value of Patient Navigation Programs

- Cynthia Cantril, Sutter Pacific Medical Foundation

Patient Navigation in a Payor Cancer Program

- Wendy Marinkovich, Blue Cross Blue Shield Association

Impact of Patient Navigation in an Integrated Care Delivery System

- Christine Valania, Geisinger Medical Center Cancer Services

Panel Discussion

10:00 am **Break**

10:15 am **Keynote Presentation**

- Greg Simon, Biden Cancer Initiative

Q&A

10:40 am Session 6: Panel Discussion: Opportunities to Advance Progress in Patient Navigation
Moderator: Karen Basen-Engquist, The University of Texas MD Anderson Cancer Center

- Tracy Battaglia, Boston University School of Medicine
- Harold P. Freeman, Harold P. Freeman Patient Navigation Institute
- Robert Green, Flatiron Health
- Linda Horn, Cancer Survivor and Former CEO, Sutter Coast Hospital

Group Discussion

11:30 am Workshop Wrap-Up
Lawrence Shulman, University of Pennsylvania
Planning Committee Co-Chair

11:45 am Adjourn